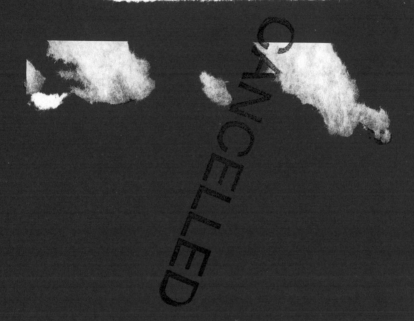

Hot
Flush

MICHELLE HEATON

Hot Flush

Motherhood, the Menopause and Me

Writing consultant Clare O'Reilly

Michael O'Mara Books Limited

First published in Great Britain in 2018
Michael O'Mara Books Limited
9 Lion Yard
Tremadoc Road
London SW4 7NQ

Copyright © Michelle Heaton 2018

A CIP catalogue record for this book is available from the British
Library.

Papers used by Michael O'Mara Books Limited are natural, recyclable
products made from wood grown in sustainable forests. The
manufacturing processes conform to the environmental regulations of
the country of origin.

ISBN: 978-1-78243-953-0 in hardback print format
ISBN: 978-1-78243-979-0 in trade paperback format
ISBN: 978-1-78243-954-7 in ebook format
ISBN: 978-1-78929-007-3 in audio book format

1 2 3 4 5 6 7 8 9 10

Design and typeset by K.DESIGN, Winscombe, Somerset

Printed and bound by CPI Group (UK) Ltd, Croydon, CRO 4YY

www.mombooks.com

Contents

I dedicate this book to my mum and dad, who raised me and my baby brother David well. You all believed in me. I also dedicate it to my superstar manager Ali, my best friend Viv and her family.

But mostly, I dedicate this book to my husband, Hugh. Without you and our two beautiful children, Faith and AJ, I'd be a broken woman. You are my rock, my best friend, and more to me than you will ever know.

Here's to the future, no more looking back …

Foreword

I've been trying to write this book for years and while I'm by no means at the end of this journey, with the toughest parts behind me and a brighter future to focus on and look forward to, it feels like the best time to commit my experiences to paper and tell the real truth about the last six years of my life. Buckle up and bear with me – it won't be easy, but it'll most definitely be honest.

When I was diagnosed with the BRCA2 gene mutation in 2012 and decided I'd be having a mastectomy with reconstructive surgery and then a hysterectomy, which would put me into surgical menopause, all I knew about the M word was that it affected older women, like my mum, who suffered hot flushes, night sweats and headaches. I thought it meant something completely different to the reality of it.

Two major surgeries later, and I've reduced my risk of breast and ovarian cancers down to a few per cent; but the emotional, physical and mental toll has been nothing short of cataclysmic, both for me and my husband and our two young children.

I'm not alone in having the faulty BRCA gene and I'm not alone in being a woman, a mother, whose life is turned upside down by something they didn't see coming and so couldn't prepare for. How we all cope with a diagnosis or change in life is very individual. I'm not saying my reactions you'll read about in the following pages are right, I'm not saying I'm proud of everything that's in this book – but it's the truth about how I coped, how my family coped, how we came close to not coping and how we eventually have learned to move forward in the face of it all.

You may have seen the TV interviews I've done or read some of the magazine stories about my experiences and the surgeries I've had, but this book lays bare the reality of what my journey has entailed. It's not sugar-coated, it doesn't fit neatly into a segment and there hasn't always been a happy ending.

It's been gut-wrenching, painful, heartbreaking, and at times it has felt impossible, but I hope my honesty about what I've been through in the last six years will change more than a few opinions on menopause and how we view the millions of women across the UK who are going through it.

I've lived a good life, one I'm incredibly thankful for; I'm a normal girl from Gateshead, I grew up on a council estate and I worked hard to get into, and stay in, the industry I'm in. I'm thirty-eight, I have a fantastic husband and great kids, and I've been blessed with wonderful friends and an amazing career. My health hasn't played ball along with the other parts of my life, but it's taught me so much about resilience, fortitude and strength, and I hope that's evident as you read through these pages.

What I also hope is apparent is that all any of us can do when faced with adversity is our best. There's no magic answer, no magic key or solution that will let us sail through the tough things life throws at us; all any of us can do is try and figure things out as we go, and learn – as much as from what doesn't work as from what does. No one knows what hand they're going to be dealt and we can all choose either to let it break us or make us.

I've had times when I've been on my knees, both literally and metaphorically, not sure whether I could get up or carry on, but in those bleak moments we can all find a reason to keep fighting. For me, that's my family, but whatever you're going through in life, find a reason to keep putting one foot in front of the other. If you can't walk, crawl, but keep moving forward: it's the only way through and at some point, a new day will begin.

At times as I went through my surgeries, I was in so much pain and hurting so much inside and out, the thought of moving forward felt impossible but, little by little, I got better, got more resilient, moved on, learned and let the experience make me a stronger woman, stronger mother, stronger friend, sister and wife.

Some of the things you'll read about in this book are things I've never told a soul and I've been honest about things that are impossibly hard to admit. At times I doubted my marriage would weather the storm, and I wouldn't have blamed my husband for walking out on me and never coming back. I'm incredibly fortunate Hugh is still my rock and while I'm committing the last six years to paper, I'm also moving on: looking forward and leaving the past that's taught me so much behind.

I'm Michelle Heaton, and this is my journey ...

CHAPTER 1

The Surgery

'I'm sorry, Michelle; it's inoperable and incurable. There's nothing we can do. While we can't be sure, you have a few weeks to get your affairs in order. I'm really very sorry…'

'Mummy, I'm hungry, I want breakfast, can I have Cheerios? Mummy?'

Jolted awake, with my heart racing, I blinked in the half light, looking around at my familiar bedroom, my Faith – all of two years old in her cute little Doc McStuffins pyjamas, scruffy blonde bedhead, eyes still half asleep – thinking about her belly and yawning while she clambered up into bed beside me. She snuggled in while I registered what had just happened, and the words I'd just heard, as clear as day.

The bedside clock swam into view – it was 5.45 a.m. I could hear my husband, Hugh, in the shower already and while everything appeared to be normal, having been startled awake, I desperately tried to process the nightmare Faith had brought me out of.

The one where I was dying.

The one where I had cancer.

The one where I'd leave my family behind.

It had a visceral reality to it I couldn't shake. In the dream, I'd been at my local hospital, the one where I'd had my preventative mastectomy and caesarean sections for Faith and my son, AJ. I'd been wearing clothes I have in my wardrobe – my turn-up, pale-blue boyfriend jeans and a coral off-the-shoulder jumper. I'd stared down at my feet, and they were in the Adidas Superstar trainers I live in when I'm not training or working. I'd been playing with the delicate gold heart necklace Hugh had bought me. I wear it round my neck and I touch it whenever I'm nervous or impatient.

I could hear the beeps of machines in other rooms and smell the hospital smell combining with Red Roses by Jo Malone, my favourite perfume. I could feel the uncomfortable back of the plastic hospital chair on my spine. While the face of the doctor hadn't been one I recognised, the manner, the official terms – it had all felt so incredibly real.

I'd been there. It had felt as real as Faith did beside me now. I'd had cancer. I'd been told I was dying.

My heart still pounding, I gathered Faith into me for a cuddle, her shallow breathing helping to regulate my still-pounding heart and calm me down. Holding her there, close to me, I tried to get to grips with the nightmare I'd just had, like somehow Faith held the key to me deciphering it and understanding it.

Breathing in the scent of her strawberry detangling shampoo and stroking the halo of her golden hair away from her face as she snuggled into me made me squeeze her that little bit tighter. I wanted to stay there in bed with her forever. If there was a time in my life I could have pressed pause at, that'd be it.

But with six-month-old AJ's cries coming from his cot, there was no way to stop the day advancing. No way to slow time. It'd tick by in seconds, minutes and hours, just like every other day.

Except this wasn't any other day.

Thursday 2 October 2014 was D Day. Or H Day, to be more accurate. I was having a hysterectomy. A procedure that would change my body irreversibly, forever. I, like 55,000 other women across the UK every year, was having an operation that would plunge me into surgical menopause and strip my body of its natural hormones.

I'd start the day as me, Michelle Heaton, a normal mum of two, and end the day without any of the organs inside me that had made my two babies possible. Right there, then, I still had the ability to have children. Holding Faith in my arms, I was exactly the same woman who'd given birth to her two years before. By the end of the day that woman would be gone forever, the ability to have my own biological children a thing of the past, and I was only in my mid-thirties – thirty-five, to be precise.

While Faith and AJ were exhausting even on their best days, a slow panic which had been rising in me for the last few days started to fight its way to the surface with increasing intensity. What if I wanted another child? What if Hugh and I decided to extend the family we were creating? Yes, AJ was only six months old and we were both exhausted because he refused to sleep past 5 a.m. most days, but what if he got to five or six and we decided we wanted more children? I was making a life-changing decision without the faintest clue of how I'd feel about it this time next week, let alone this time next year or the one after.

I'd made the decision to have my ovaries, womb and fallopian tubes removed to reduce my risk of getting ovarian cancer – the disease that had killed my paternal grandmother, Maria, after she'd battled it once already in her thirties, around the same age I was now. By the time she'd passed away in her eighties from that second bout of ovarian cancer, she had already battled breast cancer twice before, and also renal cancer.

While I'd thought and rethought my decision a hundred times over, I was still panicking that morning that it was the wrong one and that I was about to make a mistake I wouldn't be able to undo. It's not that I ever doubted it was the right thing to do – the BRCA gene mutation is one of the most serious in the world – but it just seemed so permanent.

Having had two caesarean sections in two years, I was putting myself through my third major abdominal surgery because, in my case, I had a 40 per cent risk of getting ovarian cancer (the percentage risk varies according to age of diagnosis, family background and other factors). With Hugh, my husband of four years, two-year-old Faith and six-month-old AJ to think about, I had a responsibility to them to reduce that risk and be around as long as I could.

I have the BRCA2 gene mutation or, as it's less snappily referred to, the breast cancer early onset gene 2 mutation. When BRCA genes function properly, they are supposed to produce tumour-suppressor proteins, but when there's an alteration or mutation in the BRCA1 or BRCA2 gene and it doesn't do its job, it inhibits the repair of DNA damage and raises the risk of disease. In short, people with a BRCA1 or BRCA2 gene mutation are at increased risk of their DNA damage building up and causing a normal cell to change into a cancerous cell.

Because I tested positive for the BRCA2 mutation, I had an 80 to 85 per cent risk of developing breast cancer and a 40 per cent risk of developing ovarian cancer. I also had a familial history of early onset – Maria had been in her late thirties the first time she'd battled ovarian cancer, whereas in other women with the defective BRCA2 gene, the disease might not occur until their late forties – so I was advised a full hysterectomy was the best way to eliminate as much risk as possible and take the statistical risk of cancer down from double figures to single ones.

Forty per cent might not sound like much, but if someone said you had a 40 per cent chance of winning the lottery, you'd buy a ticket, right? It was too high a number for me to opt for watchful waiting, or to leave it any longer than I had already – especially considering the fact that ovarian cancer is considered a silent killer. Over 75 per cent of cases in the UK aren't diagnosed until the cancer has spread to the abdomen, and a life expectancy of just five years after diagnosis is commonplace. I'd done my research on what I was looking at and while I'd learned the figures like a script, I was incredibly panicked at what was going to happen to me that morning.

I left Faith snuggled in bed for a second while I scooped AJ out of his cot, and then I took them both downstairs for their breakfast. While I made coffee for Hugh and fed AJ his baby porridge, I wrestled with how normal the routine felt compared to how abnormal the day would be.

My phone pinged to life with a text from my best friend, Vivianna, snapping me out of my melancholy – she was on her way to me in Hertfordshire from north London, where she lived, to look after the children. I always get excited about her impending arrival when she comes to visit; she's been my best friend for the better part of eighteen years, we lived together when I moved up to London for Liberty X and she's godmother to my children. She's quite simply one of the most amazing human beings I've ever had the fortune to know and call a friend. Seeing her always makes me smile, but that morning I knew it would mean we were one step closer to the operation. Viv had volunteered to mind the children while Hugh took me into hospital and they'd agreed to tag team while I was there; one of them with Faith and AJ and one of them with me, as long as I needed it.

With Viv on her way and leaving Hugh with the babies after his shower, I went upstairs to get myself ready. It was 6.30 a.m. and I was due at the hospital at 9 a.m. I had an hour and a half before I had to leave, and the next time I put my key in the front door, everything would be different.

I showered and changed, pulled my hair back, and applied some tinted moisturiser and a slick of lip gloss before I did a final check of my bag. I had a list on my phone I'd made, and I triple-checked the contents. Inside was a comfy bright-pink nightdress – I'd been advised not to bring pyjamas as the waistband would sit where the surgical wound would be – a couple of changes of clothes and my toiletries. With my laptop packed, some books for reading and my mobile phone charger safely stowed away too, I was my usual organised self, ready early and completely prepared.

I zipped up my bag and carried it downstairs. In spite of the rising panic, I knew nothing had been forgotten, nothing overlooked. Everything was on point, every 'i' dotted and every 't' crossed. Emotionally, however, it was a different matter. The panic I felt that morning was a culmination of thoughts from the last few months, from the day I'd booked the hysterectomy and committed it to the calendar in the kitchen. Throughout the whole run-up, I'd concentrated more on the averting the risk of cancer side of the hysterectomy than I had the emotional napalm bomb that was about to go off in my family. I had no idea then what I know now.

If I could go back to that morning, the first thing I'd do would be to sit down and have a very long chat with myself about what was about to happen. I'd speak to Hugh, and ask for tolerance and understanding, and explain we'd have a hell of a storm to weather together, and I'd remind the kids I love them with the very fibre of my being, despite what might come... But that morning, while I knew it was major surgery and I was irreversibly changing my body, I hadn't at all factored in the emotional impact I'd soon collide with.

When I'd had a double mastectomy and reconstruction to lower my risk of breast cancer two years earlier, in 2012, on the run-up to that surgery, I'd prepared myself, because I knew there'd be a physical change – something everyone could see. With this operation, while I knew I'd be going into menopause, other than adding a scar to where I had two already, externally I wouldn't look any different to how I did before the operation. With hindsight, I guess I assumed things wouldn't be that different afterwards because I wouldn't look that different. No one would know looking at me that I didn't have my own ovaries, so how different would that make me feel? I suspected, not much.

I heard Viv arrive and when I shouted down that I was on my way, I heard the kettle on and heard her laughing with Faith. It all felt so completely normal.

As I said goodbye to Viv and kissed and held the children while Hugh loaded up the car, I wondered how I'd deal with hot sweats at work or headaches like my mum had endured during her menopause. I'd spoken to Mum at length about her experience when I knew I'd be going into it in my thirties, and she'd told me all about the physical symptoms she endured. Two years of headaches at the same time every month, which no painkiller would stop or make it go away, but then as suddenly as they'd started, they'd stopped. I wondered what symptoms I'd have, how I'd cope, like Mum had.

While I knew about her journey and had done some online research, Mr Sheridan – my gynaecologist, who'd also delivered Faith and AJ – hoped hormones would control it all; that with a little trial and error we'd get to a point where everything was evened out and I'd carry on as normal. He'd explained that when my ovaries were removed I'd have an implant of oestrogen put under the skin on my bottom; it would take over where my ovaries left off and would continue to release oestrogen into my body in the absence of my ovaries. My hormone levels would go into autopilot, and it should be business as usual, with them remaining stable. The implant would need to be changed every six months, but it'd slowly release oestrogen and he was confident the physical and hormonal symptoms – which had caused so much discomfort to my mum – wouldn't plague me.

I knew it could potentially take a while for my hormone levels to sort themselves out, but I didn't factor in how many tears I'd cry while my emotional state tried to right itself. It's only with the benefit of hindsight three years later, typing these words, that I can acknowledge, admit to and try to deal with how woefully underprepared I was emotionally for what I was about to go through.

I thought it'd be like having a caesarean section, and I'd had two of those before, so I assumed I knew what I was looking at. With both Faith in 2012 and AJ in 2014 there'd been a recovery time where I was immobile and getting better, then life had gone on. I thought I was going to wake up after a hysterectomy with the flat stomach I'd gone in with, get better and everything would carry on as normal. I hadn't been told otherwise by anyone. It sounds incredibly naïve, I know that, but I'm being honest and if I can't be honest less than 4,000 words into what's been the hardest journey of my life, then when can I be?

I was in the dark about what I'd look like and what I could do post-operatively, and while it's easy to point a finger at the doctors and nurses who treated me, the reality is that I hadn't asked how I'd look after the operation. I'd had some genetic counselling at the very beginning – that's all I'd accepted – but none of it had talked about the physicality of a double mastectomy and reconstruction or the hysterectomy – which back then was just on the horizon.

I knew I'd need a recovery time; it's why I'd asked Viv to help us out as much as she could, and my mum would be coming down when I got out of hospital to help with Faith and AJ for a while when Hugh went back to work, but I thought within a few days I'd be walking fine and I'd be over it all in a few weeks maximum – back to normal, just like we were that morning. One more thing to tick off the list, and then we could move on with life without the BRCA shadow hanging over us any more.

The mastectomy two years earlier had been straightforward; I'd packed a bag, gone in to hospital, had it done, recovered, got on with it. There'd been a period post-operatively when I was sore and bandaged and had drains in, but I'd come home from hospital after a few days and while Faith had been a baby and wanted to crawl all over my chest, comparatively speaking I'd been fine and up and about again fairly fast.

I just assumed the same thing would happen with the hysterectomy. I honestly thought I might even wake up lighter because I was getting things removed from my body. I know now how daft that sounds – but I was getting three organs removed, surely by the very nature of removing them I'd lose weight? I'd weighed myself before I got in the shower that morning and had written it down on my phone to compare it with a post-operative weight. Looking back now, I can wholeheartedly appreciate how stupid my thought process was.

Mr Sheridan had talked me through the process and asked me if I wanted to see a counsellor before or afterwards, but I'd had a lot of hours with a genetic counsellor to adjust to being BRCA positive when I'd been diagnosed with it in 2012. I thought I'd had enough counselling and I didn't need any more before another operation. I didn't know then that genetic counselling, which helps inform treatment decisions, and therapeutic counselling, which helps you come to terms with the emotional impact, were so very different, so when it was offered, I felt I didn't need it.

I couldn't have been more wrong.

For anyone who's reading this, thinking, 'What's with her? How did she go into it so naïvely?' you're asking a really good question and one I've tried to answer myself too many times. Part of the answer is that I hate googling things for myself where health is concerned because I'm scared of what I'll read. Yes, I researched what I was avoiding, but I didn't want to research what I was doing, as odd as that sounds. When you find out you have a gene that could lead to cancers that can kill you, Google becomes a scary place.

The gap between finding out I had the faulty BRCA2 gene

and having the mastectomy had been terrifying enough. I'd spent hours with Faith as a baby sleeping on my chest while I read story after story about women who had it and who'd lost most of their family to it. I'd googled myself into a near hysteria after I got the results, and it put me off googling too much about my own health.

Besides, I didn't want to scare myself out of having the procedure. Having a hysterectomy would make me live longer, and that was priority number one and what I'd focused on. I hadn't searched what I'd look like afterwards or how long recovery would take because in the grand scheme of things before the operation I didn't think it'd matter. I'd be taking my risk of cancer down to a few per cent, which was far more important, wasn't it?

When Hugh drove me the 1.8 miles from home to Spire Bushey Hospital the morning of my operation, there wasn't a dreaded silence in the car, there weren't any tears. Yes, I was nervous – any general anaesthetic carries risk – but I was so underprepared that I had no idea what I was walking into. There'd been tears when I'd gone into surgery to have the mastectomy, but this was my second procedure and after this, once I'd recovered, we'd be looking at a long life together with a dramatically reduced risk of cancer.

Hugh and I were far more matter-of-fact about what we thought lay ahead because on paper, after the operation, we'd be out of the woods. I'd still have the gene but the potential for it to cause cancer would be almost completely gone.

Having parked up, we checked in and I was shown to my room; Hugh had made sure I was comfortable and okay after I was prepped for surgery, then he kissed me goodbye and told me he loved me.

'I love you too, Hugh, kiss the kids for me and I'll see you on the other side.'

That was it.

No tears.

No trauma.

No trouble.

As the anaesthetic went in, I started counting backwards from ten.

A countdown to a completely different me.

I thought the minute I woke up I'd feel empty where the potentially cancer-causing organs had been taken away. I'd been sure emptiness would be the most immediate physical difference when I came to and while I felt nothing like the woman who'd started counting backwards from ten, my presumption couldn't have been further from the truth.

Eight hours after Hugh left my side, as the lights and the room swam into view, I could feel someone holding my hand. The familiar long fingers, the wedding ring I'd put on his left hand in the Bahamas four years earlier grew clearer, and the soft Dublin accent I loved with all my heart whispered, 'Do you feel any different? Are you OK? I love you...'

My mouth dry and a quick scan of the room to make sure no little ears could hear me, all I was able to utter was, 'No, I just feel fucking sore. I'm just sore. I'm in pain, Hugh. It really, really hurts...'

I was dosed up with tramadol – an opioid pain medication – but the agony was still searing through my abdomen. I thought I'd feel like I'd had a caesarean section and while it felt similar in some ways, I was in much more pain than I had been after the caesarean sections that had delivered me my babies. The soreness, not being able to move, the catheter, the drains in my stomach, the painkillers they'd given me, the beeps from the machines, everything seemed to hurt way more.

I was shocked and panicked.

I was even more sedated than after a caesarean section, but everything felt horrendous. Anyone who's had a caesarean section will know you remember more about your children arriving than you do about the pain, but a hysterectomy is a different animal altogether. Now I had nothing except pain, and the chance of ever having another baby was gone completely and irreversibly. Forever.

In so many ways the physical feeling I was dealing with reminded me of my babies but it made the fact I could never have biological ones again even harder to deal with. Feeling the same way but without that prize plunged me instantly into depression. I felt tearful and emotional, like all the fears I'd been battling all morning and in the weeks running up to today had been confirmed. I closed my eyes, longing to be back in bed next to Faith asking for her Cheerios, but when I opened them again, I was still in a hospital bed.

It was late, and I was beyond groggy, too groggy to try and explain the thoughts, half-thoughts and disconnected trails of sentences that were swimming around my opioid-addled head. Hugh shushed me back to sleep and told me he'd be there with me, holding my hand. After he sat with me for a while as I slept, drifting in and out of sedated state, he kissed my forehead and squeezed my hand, whispering he'd be back in the morning with Faith, who wanted to see Mummy.

I slept like a baby that night. I was groggy from surgery and the nurses kept my pain medication topped up, so while any movement hurt like hell, I was pretty medicated and don't remember much about my first night post surgery. I missed the children but my body and my mind were exhausted. I was uncomfortable and in pain, but I managed to get a decent amount of rest.

The second day, though, was one of the worst of my life.

I woke up alone, feeling instantly emotional about what I'd done and what had been taken away from me. In pain, I felt the most homesick I've ever felt and longed to be back in my bed with Faith and AJ beside me. I knew from pre-surgical consultations that day two would be the day they'd get me to stand up – supported by nurses, of course. It had been the hardest part of the caesarean sections I'd had, so I knew what I was heading for, but it felt ten times worse than it had when I'd had Faith and AJ. I didn't want to try and stand, I wanted to stay in bed and curl up and make it all go away.

My medical team had other ideas though. As the nurses stood by my bed, preparing to help me up, Hugh texted to say he was on his way in with Faith and would arrive in ten minutes. The nurses had made me drink lots of water and as they took the catheter out for my first wee, I thought I'd collapse in agony. I had a drainage tube in my belly and I gagged at the pain searing through my abdomen as I felt it move deep inside my wound.

As I gently stood for the first time in menopause, I caught sight of my reflection in the mirror and gasped. I was so dizzy, I had to blink a few times to check the reflection looking back at me was actually mine and not someone else's. My face showing all the pain I felt, devastation swept over me.

I felt and looked terrible.

I had what looked like the belly of a pregnant lady and I was hunched like a woman in her eighties. I looked puffy and bloated, nothing like I thought I would. The last time I'd undergone abdominal surgery, I'd been smiling from ear to ear with AJ in my arms, exhausted but rosy-cheeked and happy. The reflection I saw now looked old, exhausted and pale, despite only having returned from a week spent in the sunshine of Las Vegas a few days before.

For the last six months I'd been working hard to get into shape post AJ, and because of my lack of mental or emotional preparation for this surgery, I was devastated by what I saw.

It. Was. The. Worst. Moment.

All the hard work I'd put into getting my body into shape had disappeared. Staring at myself, there wasn't a single part of me that looked anything like the Michelle Heaton who'd gone in for the surgery just twenty-four hours previously. Not even my face.

The nurses slowly helped me take the baby steps I needed to get to the toilet in my room and while they showed me the cord to pull if I needed them, they said they'd slip out while I was on the toilet. They'd come back in a few minutes to help me get back into bed.

I sat on the toilet in agony, my head spinning at the memory of the reflection I'd caught sight of. Weeing was excruciating, but my mind was racing. I heard the door open, thinking the nurses had come back to help me into bed again, but when Faith's familiar call of 'Mummy' came echoing through the open toilet door, the tears started to fall.

'Hugh, no, don't bring her in, I don't want ...'

'Mummy?'

'Hugh? No! Please.'

I shouted this time. I couldn't move to shut the door and I was terrified my beautiful daughter's little face would peer round the corner any time.

Children can't lie, and Faith is an open book of emotion – whatever she's thinking, you can see on her face, and I knew my reflection would shock her. She wouldn't be able to disguise it and while I didn't want to scare her, I also knew she'd make me feel even worse than I already did because she'd confirm what I knew already – that I looked nothing like the woman who'd gone in for the surgery.

There was an urgency to my voice which Hugh caught, and I saw him ushering Faith behind his long legs, shielding her from the view of her mummy hunched over on the toilet, sobbing.

'Shell, it's fine, she's desperate to see you...'

'Hugh, get her out of here, I can't see her, I don't want either of you to see me like this. Just go. Go... GO!' I was shouting. Loud, and for someone who sings for a career, I can shout pretty loudly.

Whether he took heed or whether he was worried I'd burst the staples holding my wound together by shouting, I don't know, but Hugh ushered a now crying Faith out the room. As I heard her sobs in the hallway, I was wracked with even louder ones.

I sobbed until I couldn't breathe and when the nurses came back into the room after Hugh left, I asked them to leave me alone for a few more minutes. They could see my tears, but I assured them I was fine, that it was just painful trying to wee for the first time since the catheter. With their concerns assuaged, they agreed to give me a few more minutes and closed the door. My tears just kept falling. I cried for the way

I'd treated my two-year-old daughter, I cried for the way I felt, the way I looked. I cried for the Michelle of yesterday and I cried for the Michelle of tomorrow and the future. Sitting there, tubes in me and the harsh hospital lights shining down on me, I sobbed tears of misery for everything: for BRCA2, for my mastectomy and for my hysterectomy. For the fact I'd never, ever be the same woman again.

As my sobs subsided to sniffs and whimpers, the nurses came in and gently ushered me to bed. They tried to make me feel better, telling me I was post-operative and would start to feel better in a few days, that it was completely normal to feel this way after such a big procedure, especially at my age, but I barely heard anything they said, much less heeded it. I was emotionally exhausted from the exchange with Faith and Hugh, and all I could do was stare into the middle distance while I tried to come to terms with it all.

Hugh texted to say he was taking Faith home and would be back in an hour. I texted him back to tell her I was sorry, that I loved her and that I missed her. I was still struggling to keep the tears in check, and they started flowing freely again when he arrived alone an hour later.

When he walked in the door, he was holding a little blue box. He couldn't hold my gaze for more than a couple of seconds before breaking away. He wasn't angry with me, but I could see how devastated he felt that both Faith and I had been in floods of tears – especially when he knew how much we loved each other – and he'd been powerless to make either of us feel better.

'Shell, the whole reason Faith came and was so desperate to see you is because of this… She wanted to give you this…'

He trailed off, his eyes looking at the floor.

I felt my face crease as the tears started streaming harder.

My little Faith had only wanted to give Mummy a Tiffany necklace with a heart on. Hugh had taken her shopping, she'd picked it out herself and had been so excited to give it to me, to see how I reacted to the special present she'd chosen for me, with its beautiful white bow. She'd done nothing wrong. She'd been her usual thoughtful, compassionate little self and I'd screamed at her to get out.

A tsunami of guilt overwhelmed me as I struggled for air while the tears ran down my face. Hugh held me as best he could, carefully moving his arms around the drains in my wound while I sobbed, and as the tears turned to sniffs he reassured me Faith was fine and would be back in later with another surprise for me.

He'd explained to her on the way home that Mummy had been in pain and having her first wee, so she'd been a little bit hurty and upset. Faith had taken him at face value and – according to him – was already excited to come in and see me later and find out whether my first wee-wee had been a success.

As usual, Hugh was able to reassure me that everything would be OK, that Faith would forgive me and that we could move on from what happened. As he tried to gently manoeuvre me from guilt to happiness at the prospect of seeing her later, our conversation moved from the incident that morning to the surgery I'd undergone just twenty-four hours before.

'I look pregnant, Hugh…' I trailed off, looking down at my swollen abdomen.

'Of course you'll look swollen,' he replied, following my gaze down my body. 'You've just had an operation, Shell. It'll take time to go down. Besides, that's the last thing you should be thinking about. Who cares how you look? You've just had a major abdominal surgery to avoid a cancer that could potentially have killed you, and left me without a wife and the kids without a mother. You need to get healthy, you need to get well, I don't care how you look. Recovery is what matters now.'

'Hugh, I don't even look like myself, I feel so different, everything hurts, and I look old and pale and hunched and tired... What's happened to me? What's gone on?'

'Shell, you're overreacting – you look tired because you've had surgery. It's a big deal, but don't start thinking there's more to it than there is. You'll be back to yourself in no time, honestly...'

'I don't think I will, Hugh. I know I only had the operation yesterday, but I don't think I'll ever be me again, everything feels awful.'

He kept trying to make me feel better, to put it all into a context where I'd get better and things would be back to normal, but every time I looked down at my body I felt a panic I couldn't explain.

A nurse who was checking my charts at the foot of the bed interjected.

'It's natural to look like that after the surgery,' she said, trying to be reassuring, but she could see by the look of devastation on my face her words weren't doing the job of soothing me as she'd intended. 'It'll take a few months to go down,' she added, attempting further to allay what she could see was a rising panic in me.

'I'm sorry, what?'

Although I was still in agony, I tried to shuffle further up the bed, as if sitting up more would change things.

'It's going to take time for the swelling from the surgery to reduce and it might not ever go away completely…'

Noting the incredulous blinking and searching for words I was doing, she leapt in again before I could utter anything.

'Of course, everyone is different. I'll give you two a few minutes and go and get you some water.'

As she slipped out, I lay my head back on the pillow. It was swimming with the words she'd just said.

'Why the fuck did nobody tell me, Hugh? You might not care how I look, but I do.'

'Shell, calm down, you're not even a full day post surgery yet, you need to relax and wait and see what happens. Honestly, Michelle, you're working at a million miles an hour and thinking too far ahead. Right now, you need to calm down, relax, rest, sleep and focus on getting better, so we can get you home and Faith and AJ can have Mummy back. Viv is coming in later to see you, so try and focus on the positive right now, OK?'

I was reeling.

I hadn't thought longer term about the reflection staring back at me; before she spoke I'd been upset in the here and now, but her words floored me. I was desperately trying to come to terms with what I'd just been told and reframe my thinking to cope with the fact I could look like this for months, possibly years or even forever.

Both in that moment and writing this now, it seems unbelievable that I hadn't thought to ask how I'd look physically post-operatively, but every woman is different and we're all different sizes and shapes when we go in for procedures, so there's no definitive answer anyway. Even if I had asked what I'd look like after the surgery, no one would have been able to tell me for sure.

While there was nothing Hugh could do to change anything, I pleaded with him anyway. 'What am I going to do, Hugh? Look at me. I'm supposed to have some TV work and a photo shoot next week! I look pregnant. I look bloody pregnant...'

The jumbled confusion in my head tumbled out as a clutter of words and disconnected thoughts in my attempt to think things through fast and come up with solutions which would stop me feeling as awful as I did about my reflection and not let anyone down at work. All Hugh could do was repeat his pep talk about how I'd recover and be fine and go back to normal, while he stroked my hand and my hair, and told me he loved me and that we'd be OK and get through it together.

In the time alone that afternoon between Hugh leaving and Viv arriving, I tried desperately not to think about anything. I wanted to sleep; I figured it could make me feel a bit brighter and I might not look as old and haggard if I rested.

I was resting and trying to relax when I heard a familiar tap of nails on the door of my room. Viv's smiling face peeked round the door, checking she had the right room. I scoured her reflection to see if she'd flinch at the Michelle that greeted her, but she showed no sign of shock or disgust and bowled in, taking a seat in the chair Hugh had vacated an hour earlier and giving my hand and arm a supportive and loving squeeze. It was all I needed, and the smile I'd plastered on to greet her slipped and my face crumpled with yet more tears.

'Shell, what's the matter? Are you OK? Do you want me to get a nurse?'

'Viv, look at me, I look awful, I feel horrendous. What have I done?'

Pushing her glasses up her nose, my best friend kissed my hand and the straight-talking I've always loved came pouring out thick and fast.

'Hugh told me you're feeling a bit shit about your reflection and the way you look, but buck up and shut up. You haven't got cancer, you're not dying, you've done this to be around for Hugh and those babies for longer. You're not sick, and the swelling will go down and you will get back to normal.'

I took a deep breath and tried to believe everything she'd said. I knew she was partly right, but I still felt terrible. 'I look awful and the scar is a big one, right where the other two were. I look terrible, I'm worried Hugh thinks so too but won't tell me. What if he goes off me, what if he doesn't fancy me any more because of what I've had done? Viv, I'm so worried and scared...'

Viv's never been one to sugar-coat anything. I've always loved her honesty and she's always known I can take whatever she's going to say – her honesty isn't always easy to hear but it comes from a good, big heart and it's always meant with the best of intentions.

'Shell, you guys have been married a few years, your relationship is incredibly strong, look at everything you've been through.'

'Yeah but now, as well as my boobs not being my own, my belly's bloated and all my ovaries and stuff are gone, and all I've got to show for it is a big belly and a big scar.'

'Shell, your tits weren't that great anyway, you've got a much nicer pair now and, besides, long-lasting relationships aren't based on physical attraction alone, they're based on something much deeper than that, and that's what you and Hugh have in droves.'

I laughed through the sniffling at her honesty about my new boobs – it was something she'd told me before, in the run-up to the mastectomy. I squeezed her hand as the nurse came in, telling us she'd be back in a few minutes to take a lunch order for me.

'Shell, I'm starving, I say we have a proper carb fest and we'll talk everything through over some refined carbs, sound like a plan?'

Viv handed me a tissue as she filled out the lunch card, and with more sandwiches, jacket potatoes and crisps than two normal women could eat in one sitting, my best friend spent the afternoon talking everything through with me. There were more tears, then Viv would say something that would make me feel resilient, only for me to start sobbing again a few minutes later. One second I'd feel OK and the next I'd be in floods.

I spent four days after surgery wondering whether the continual waves of tears were the onset of the emotional roller coaster of menopause or whether they were just Michelle crying because she hadn't prepared herself enough for how she'd look after having a hysterectomy. The truth is I'll never know.

I hate not having a plan or a way to make things right when they go wrong, and I was woefully unprepared for all those post-surgery feelings. So despite my mind racing, I had nothing: no thoughts, no ideas, no plan, no way to fix it. I just felt overwhelmed with panic, devastation and heartbreak.

Anyone reading this who thinks it's a self-absorbed way to think, before you judge, let me try to explain. I know I was reducing my risk of several different types of cancer and I know that the surgery – while physically different to what I expected post-operatively – would potentially give me many more years with my family. I got all of that, but I'd expected that, so there wasn't a euphoric high from that knowledge. What is difficult to come to terms with is that, whichever way I tried to cut it mentally, I was in a world of physical pain and dealing with an emotional fallout I hadn't expected, all for what was ultimately a 'maybe'.

That's what continues to be so hard about the path I chose to this very day, and it's something lots of women who have the BRCA mutation will identify with; they tell me about it when I meet them too, so I know I'm not alone. When I put myself through a mastectomy and reconstructive surgery and the hysterectomy that plunged me into surgical menopause, I didn't have cancer. I don't have cancer now, I have a gene that could *cause* cancer, and they're two very different things. I've spoken to women in their seventies who have the faulty BRCA gene and have never had cancer, and I've read of women in their twenties who had it and passed away from ovarian cancer. I opted to have two very invasive sets of preventative surgery, and while I'll always be glad I erred on the side of caution, there's no avoiding or ignoring the fact I could have reached my grave with my body intact and no cancer.

How I look and my appearance are a huge part of what's made my career and, believe me, I know how that sounds. Maybe if I was a rocket scientist, an engineer or a surgeon, my self-worth and confidence would come from my brain, or what I could do with my hands, but singing, dancing, acting and presenting are what I do for a living, and you don't get the roles if you don't look right. I work in an industry that judges on appearance, so the prospect of looking like I did post-operatively had huge implications on my entire life.

After my carb fest with Viv, she left me and went to swap places with Hugh again. While I tried to rest, I couldn't help but wonder what would happen to my career if I never looked like my pre-operative self again. Hugh came back later that afternoon with Faith in a Doc McStuffins outfit. She'd come to the conclusion that Mummy needed Faith to make her well again and she'd begged Hugh to buy her one, complete with a little plastic doctor's case.

I heard her little feet running down the hallway before she entered the room. She'd forgotten the morning's trauma and was as delighted to see me as ever. She clambered on my bed and, being mindful of my staples, she listened to my heart with her little plastic stethoscope, pretending to fix Mummy and make her better, while I stroked her hair and cuddled her as best I could. In addition to the drains coming out my stomach, I had a drip in my arm and a pulse measure on my finger, so with all the wires it was difficult for her to get as close as I desperately wanted her to, but we persevered.

I was exhausted and on tramadol, and while she babbled on endlessly about what Daddy had done her for tea last night, what Viv had done for breakfast and what AJ had been up to, I whispered I was sorry. And with her big heart and endless forgiveness, my little Faith kissed me and told me it didn't matter.

We spent the afternoon together, her playing with the brand-new necklace she'd bought me, and with her little arms around me and her little hands on my new necklace, I felt the first bit of calm I'd felt since coming round from the anaesthetic. It was a brief moment of respite from what was, in the first few days after the operation, an emotional ground zero. I'd cry while I was alone but then try and be brave for

Hugh and Faith. I'd tell myself I could get back into shape, I'd done it twice after the children, surely I could do it again? But every glimpse of my hunched reflection made me feel like I'd never be the same again.

I also felt like somehow I wasn't really dealing with the underlying reason for the tears which kept coming; yes, I hated my reflection, but it felt like there was something bigger I was mourning for. But, try as I might, I couldn't make sense of it. I knew what needed to be done to fix how I looked and how I felt; gym sessions are always my tonic, but moving gently in bed was still agony. I knew I was months away from being able to hit the gym like I wanted to, and I think that added to a growing frustration I was feeling.

I spent the next three nights before discharge constantly trying to remind myself I'd gone through all this in order to be around longer for my family, but the reality was that I'd swing between tears of pain and tears for the long road of physical recovery I had ahead of me. I felt unprepared for everything, and nothing I did helped me catch up on that feeling, change it or get ahead of it. I googled lots about recovery times and how physically I'd change in the weeks and months of recovery to come, but it felt like a seismic shift had happened and I couldn't figure it out no matter how hard I tried.

I felt and looked like I'd aged thirty years in only a few days in hospital. Hugh was adamant I didn't look like I thought I did, so was it psychological? I don't know; Hugh would reassure me daily I didn't look any different but my reflection – or at least what I thought I saw when I looked in the mirror – told me otherwise. I didn't have any oomph. I felt like I lost my sparkle, I was terrified I'd never be the woman who'd gone under general anaesthetic again. I'd woken up feeling only 80 per cent me, and that figure didn't change when I was released from hospital four days later.

My Menopause Musings

With hindsight, maybe I'd have waited a little while longer before putting my body and my family through what I have, but I know having the surgery was the right thing to do, even if I was woefully underprepared for it.

Ovarian cancer is very hard to detect; symptoms are similar to lots of other things, like your time of the month, a urinary tract infection or IBS, which often means by the time it's diagnosed, it's too late and the fight for survival is on. Take into consideration the fact my gran had it when she was so young, not to mention the fact my great-grandmother had battled ovarian and breast cancer too, deep down I never doubted I'd done the right thing, even though I struggled after the operation.

I don't want to deter women from going through with it, because it hasn't been the worst thing in my life. The worst thing in my life would be getting ovarian cancer. The worst thing for me would be to continue to live knowing the BRCA2 gene mutation was a ticking time bomb in my body, which could go off at any time. But I do know I should have asked for more counselling. When it felt like the wheels were coming off my wagon in those early days, I should have told one of the nurses, explained to my doctor I was struggling to hold myself together, that I was confused and scared and didn't know what I was feeling. Putting a brave face on it was without a doubt the wrong thing to do.

I'd have also prepared myself for the physical difference too. Because I was so woefully underprepared for that part of it, I was mentally scarred for a long time by what I saw and what I felt, both of which I'm still coming to terms with now.

For anyone who's about to embark on this journey, or is considering it, or has just had it done, keep some kind of journal or diary. Whether you have the BRCA gene mutation, are in early menopause or are about to undergo surgical menopause, record your feelings and emotions on the run-up and during it, and I promise it will help you. I didn't, and I wish I had. If I'd been able to keep a track of those waves of emotion, they'd maybe have been less scary. Having a space to unburden myself, as well as to have a document of my experience, would have been incredibly emotionally beneficial in my recovery. It might have helped me identify emotional triggers, search for developing patterns of behaviour. It would have let me see whether I was growing more resilient day by day or whether I wasn't; either way it would have been useful.

I've thought long and hard about the things I wish I'd known about the hysterectomy going into it. They might not be the same for everyone, but if I'd known these five things ahead of time, my recovery might not have been such a shock or so difficult.

1) You won't wake up slimmer

Yes, you're getting organs removed and, yes, it's major abdominal surgery. Be prepared to wake up looking pregnant, not slimmer than when you went in. You'll be bloated and hunched but while your posture might look terrible to begin with, it won't last.

2) You will wake up (and stay) exhausted

A hysterectomy is like no other procedure. It's major abdominal surgery without the joy of a newborn. Any surgery carries fatigue as a side effect of healing. A 2002 study found women felt fatigued for up to ten weeks post surgery, with a third of those surveyed still exhausted six months after the procedure. The choices of post-surgical hormone replacement therapy (HRT) and treatment are vast but, whatever you choose, don't fight the exhaustion. It's normal. Rest. You'll wake up different but don't be afraid, you'll get back to who you are and if you're finding it that hard to cope, speak to someone. Reach out and ask for help. It's there and counselling is available should you need it, so make the most of it and don't try and go it alone.

3) Number twos don't come easy

While my first wee was emotionally and physically exhausting because of what happened with Faith, my first proper toilet trip wasn't any easier. I was given stool softeners and drank plenty of water, but while I urinated the day after the operation when my catheter came out, a number two was much harder to come by. Don't stress though, it'll happen.

4) Burping, standing, farting, sneezing, laughing and leaning will be agony

Any bodily function or command that involves any effort from your abdomen or any organs close by will be agony in the first few weeks. I thought I'd burst my wound with my first post-surgery sneeze.

5) You're not alone

Ask whatever questions you want or need answers to. You're not expected to come through this unscathed, so don't pretend you are. There are occupational therapists, doctors, nurses, physiotherapists – use their expertise as much as you need. Only by arming yourself with as much knowledge as you can muster will you be able to start to come to terms with menopause and what it might mean for your future. Don't be afraid of being scared and vulnerable, it's normal.

CHAPTER 2

The Shock of BRCA: Life-changing News and my Baby Girl

I was seven months pregnant with Faith in November 2011 when my home phone rang with a familiar 0191 number. My dad, Chris, was delighted about the impending arrival of his first grandchild and would check in all the time to see how I was doing. He had only been back in my life a few months and things were still a bit awkward between us, try as we might to gloss over it. He'd walked out on my mum, Christine, just four years before: in early 2007, after almost thirty years of marriage.

The fallout was massive – it felt like it came out of the blue, although, looking back, neither of them had been their happiest for as long as I could remember. But Mum hadn't seen it coming and had settled for the fact they'd be together for the rest of their lives, and it was a huge shock to the whole family. They'd spent almost thirty years bringing myself and my brother David up; we'd been the distraction for years between them that meant they didn't have to face up to the fact their happily ever after had disintegrated, but since we'd left home, the years hadn't been kind to either of them. They'd ended up existing rather than really living and loving together. With us no longer living at home, they'd had no choice but to focus on themselves rather than their children.

Dad being the one who'd made the decision to change things and leave my mum, I'd sided with her. I'd had a nagging feeling for years that she'd given everything up to be with him and I'd found out I was right. They'd met in the navy, and when they left it was Dad who progressed into other careers. She'd built a home and a life for us all, but had put herself on the bottom of her list of priorities. She'd selflessly given up the best years of her life to be a mum and a wife, and when Dad left her, she didn't know what to do. She didn't know how to pay a bill, change a mortgage rate, sort the TV licence; Dad had done all that for her while she'd raised a family and kept the home and worked part-time too. When he went, I took over the role of being dad and I resented him for that. I became the husband to Mum – confidante, carer and supporter. I didn't hate Dad as a person, but I hated the position he put me in.

Thinking he was being selfish, I cut him out of my life and he'd moved on with someone else. But when his mum, my grandmother, Maria passed away in January 2010, we'd met again at her funeral – the first time he'd met my Hugh. Maria had died of a broken heart after her husband John, my step-granddad, passed away the previous July. Having battled cancer four times already, the fifth diagnosis, a secondary bout of ovarian cancer which was terminal, had been too much to bear. She'd decided eighty-nine was a long enough innings for her, and she wanted out of life. While Dad and I still had a lot of ground to make up, we'd grown slowly closer since Maria's passing.

Like always when he phoned that Thursday in November, we went through the small talk, him asking about my pregnancy, how I was feeling, when my next scan was and whether I'd decided on a name; me asking how he was keeping, what he'd been up to and what the weather was like in my home town of Gateshead. We chatted about David's latest antics in Australia and where he was going next, and what we both had on workwise in the coming weeks.

During the first lull in the conversation, he took the opportunity to tell me something that would change the course of my life forever.

'Tuppence, there's something I need to tell you about.'

Tuppence had been my nickname when I was little; whenever I did well in a singing or dancing competition, he'd hug me tight and say, 'I'm proud of you, Tuppence, well done.' Mum never called me it and Dad had never called David by the name, it was ours alone. I'd loved the nickname as a little girl, when it came out I knew Dad was especially pleased with me, and while it might have sounded like a pet name, I knew it was his way of telling me he loved me. He still calls me it on texts and emails to this day, despite the fact I'm thirty-eight. But when he called me by my usual name on that grey Thursday, I had no idea that what he'd tell me next would not only shape the rest of my life but also potentially that of the daughter growing safe and warm in my pregnant belly.

He took a deep breath and explained that the ovarian cancer that had recurred in Maria before she died was a genetic type of cancer. He said he was being tested to see if he carried the gene mutation that had caused it. Maria had tested positive for the gene mutation before she died and having had a mother who'd also had breast cancer when she was young, there was reason to believe genetics played a part in both their cancers. Dad explained he'd be having a blood test and he'd know the results in a few weeks.

'What does that mean for you?' was my reply when he stopped talking. I didn't for one second think about me. Not. Once.

He explained if he had the gene he'd be at a heightened risk for testicular cancer, prostate cancer and melanoma and that, should he get a positive result, there was a 50:50 chance both my brother David and I might too.

It didn't feel like a cataclysmic phone call that would forever alter the direction of the rest of my life. I didn't hang up and write a will, check the life insurance or crumple into a heap. My heart didn't skip a beat, my voice didn't catch in my throat and my head didn't start to spin. The conversation was one of the most pedestrian we've ever had, to the point that I can't even remember much else about it.

He didn't mention BRCA2, and back then Angelina Jolie was a movie star, not a BRCA gene ambassador. Sharon Osbourne was the woman married to Ozzy and an *X Factor* judge, not the woman who carried a potentially fatal gene. BRCA didn't mean then what it does now, so even if he'd told me the name of the gene, it wouldn't have meant any more to me. Only in 1993 did scientists identify the region of the human genome in which the BRCA gene is located. In 1994 that region was narrowed down further, and BRCA1 was eventually identified. It wasn't until the end of 1995 that the BRCA2 gene was identified and only in the last five years – a year or so after I found out I had the gene – has the full significance of it reached the mainstream media and the headlines.

There are cancer-causing genes identified every year and while BRCA is now a gene the majority of people have heard of, since 2003, eight more breast cancer-causing genes have been identified, including one cancer-accelerating oncogene which could be responsible for over 4,000 cases of breast cancer in the UK every year.

While that's all a bit sciencey, it should give you an idea of how a genetic diagnosis like that back then just simply didn't mean what it does now. I didn't even think about the conversation with Dad until he phoned a few weeks later. I didn't call him the day of the screening and I hadn't bothered to ask what day he was going to get the results or whether anyone would be there to go with him.

When he called, I thought it was for his regular catch-up, but it wasn't.

This time no small talk, just tears.

The results were positive.

He carried the gene and as he cried down the phone to me from 269 miles away, I didn't know what to say to him. Dad never shared much emotion, never talked about how he felt, he was pretty much always on an even keel. I'd seen him cry a few times in my life, but he was never comfortable with that level of emotion. It was like the tears would catch him off guard; he'd bottle everything up until the dam broke and the tears would flow, but he'd shore up the dam again as quickly as possible and pretend it hadn't happened.

It sounds unkind, but I hated him crying. It always unsettled me and does to this day. Who likes to hear their daddy cry? No one, and I hated the feeling that I couldn't fix his distress. So when his upset echoed down the phone, it unnerved me the way it used to when I was a kid.

As he tried to stop the tears flowing, he reiterated what it could mean for David and me, telling me it was more serious for females to have the BRCA2 gene as the risks of ovarian and breast cancer were much higher than the risks for testicular cancer in men. He didn't give me any figures, but he was adamant I should get tested, reminding me that Maria had been young when she'd been diagnosed with both breast and ovarian cancer. He was going to try and get hold of David in Australia to tell him, but he wanted me to be the first person he told because of the weight of what it could mean for me.

Despite my platitudes to try and calm him down, he kept apologising; he seemed panicked by the prospect that there was a 50:50 chance he'd passed it on to me, but back then I hadn't spoken to a geneticist, much less googled the four letters and one number that would change everything.

I had no idea his sobs might be warranted, and I thought he was overreacting and being overly emotional for no reason. I didn't know how sinister the gene could be, didn't realise I had something that could trigger a silent killer in me. I took what he told me at face value and while he tried to stress his concerns and worries for me, I honestly believed that it meant something for him more than it meant something for me. Despite him telling me my equal odds of having the gene abnormality, because he seemed so upset about his result, I worried about him and how he felt rather than how it affected me.

It's only now I realise he was upset at passing it on to me, not the fact that he had it himself. After all, I didn't have cancer, I'd never found any lumps or bumps in my breasts, I'd attended every cervical screening I'd been invited to and all had been fine. Besides, I was pregnant and had been scanned, surely they'd have found something sinister if it existed?

His tears seemed utterly unwarranted then.

In the years since that phone call I've cried a sea of tears for Faith and for AJ in exactly the same way he did for me that day. I've been wracked with the same guilt he felt on that call, I've blamed myself for the fact I could have passed a defective gene on to them that could end their lives prematurely or at the very least put them in the position where they might have to have elective preventative surgeries. But back then I didn't know anything that I know now.

When his tears and apologies subsided, he told me I'd be getting a letter through the post inviting me to be screened for the gene mutation he carried. He wanted me to promise that I'd get tested and take it seriously. We knew three generations of our family on his side had had the BRCA2 abnormality already. I'd be invited to take the test and see if I had it. David would get the same letter and it'd be up to us whether we decided to go ahead with genetic testing or whether we preferred to live in blissful ignorance about a potential genetic time bomb inside us both.

The BRCA gene becomes more penetrant with age, which means the longer you live with the faulty gene without taking action, the higher the risk of you developing cancer. BRCA isn't related to an increased risk in any childhood cancers but as those women and men who have tested positive age, the odds shorten and the risk becomes higher.

I was thirty-two and had already lived into my thirties with it, despite there being up to an 85 per cent risk of me developing cancer. With hindsight, and knowing what I know now about the BRCA gene, my ignorance seems astounding. But back then I honestly thought Dad was overreacting, after all I'd made it this far fine – there was nothing that had happened, no health scares or ailments or symptoms I'd had which would suggest I had it, so what was the huge panic about? I ended the call by promising him I'd take it seriously, but after hanging up and worrying about him for a few minutes, it didn't really enter my head again.

With a pregnancy in progress and new baby to plan for, work and a nursery to decorate, Dad's call only came back into my mind when an innocuous white envelope landed on my doormat a few weeks later. The postmark was from the Centre for Life in Newcastle. As Dad had anticipated, I was invited to screen for the BRCA2 gene mutation.

Invited.

The only thing I really recall about opening the letter was how odd 'invited' seemed to be in that context. It wasn't a party, a launch event, an awards ceremony. Those are things to be 'invited' to, not a blood test which will tell you whether you have a faulty gene or not.

I put the letter away, adding it to my mental list of things to get done at some point.

Two weeks before she was due to be brought into the world via caesarean section, less than six weeks after the letter arrived on my doormat, Faith Michelle Hanley decided she'd had enough of waiting and my waters broke at 2 a.m. She was born at 8.15 a.m. on 11 January 2012. She was 7lb 5oz of perfect, and I was overwhelmed with love for her instantly, in awe of what Hugh and I had been able to create and what my body had been able to nurture.

I was diagnosed with arrhythmia, an irregular heartbeat, when I was twenty-five after abusing diet pills from the age of nineteen. I've given myself a long-term heart condition thanks to an ephedrine addiction, which was diagnosed in 2004 when Liberty X were at the height of their fame. I've had to wear a loop recorder to monitor my heart rate for over two years from 2012 to 2014, which has left a scar on my chest, and I've been told I'll need a pacemaker at some point in my life.

Arrhythmia is something I have and although it doesn't own me, with the attacks unpredictable, my pregnancy consultant decided a caesarean section for Faith would be safer. But my daughter decided not to wait and after a mad dash to the hospital she was born via an emergency caesarean section. Thankfully I'm a planner and always ready for things well ahead of time, so my bag was already packed when my waters broke in the middle of the night. Faith's birth – while dramatic, like she'd grow up to be – remains one of the best moments of my entire life.

So, to say the conversation I'd had with Dad was at the back of my mind when she was born is an understatement. I hadn't thought about it at all since filing the letter away in the drawer and with my baby daughter in my arms, I was fully focused on looking forward, no idea how quickly I'd be forced to look back.

I'd decided before Faith was born I'd donate her cord blood to help with medical research; it just seemed like the right thing to do and the hospital she was being born at offered the service. With her cord safely stored and ready for transportation to the donation unit, I was given a form to fill in by one of the nurses to detail my medical history and the history of both Hugh's family and mine too.

So far, so straightforward.

I was able to answer everything except for whether there was a genetic link to any illnesses or conditions in my family.

Dad's revelation surfaced somewhere in my mind, and I asked Hugh what I should say.

'He told me the name of the gene, it's some initials beginning with B, he's really worried I have it and I have the letter at home, but I haven't made the appointment yet. I thought I'd wait until I had Faith and then try and get round to it on maternity leave...'

I trailed off because I could see one of the nurses in the room looking at me and listening to what I'd whispered to Hugh. She apologised profusely for eavesdropping but asked me to elaborate, as she thought she might be able to help. I explained Dad's positive genetic test and the fact he was the third generation of our family to have a cancer-causing gene which had killed previous female members of our family.

She asked if it was the BRCA gene and on hearing the letters in the right order I was able to confirm it was. She explained the BRCA2 gene mutation was in her family too and that she'd been tested and had been negative. She wasn't lecturing me, she simply reiterated what Dad had said, that it carried an increased risk of female-specific cancers, including ovarian cancer, and that she was really glad she'd been tested and hugely relieved to find out she didn't have the gene.

The next ten words sent me into a tailspin in a way Dad's phone calls hadn't.

'You've just had a little girl; she could have it.'

She went on to connect the dots in a way I hadn't until that point. Dad had it, ergo there was a 50:50 chance I had it and if I did have it, there was also a 50:50 chance I'd passed it on to Faith, who wasn't even an hour old.

The thought that if I had it – this gene defect that caused breast and ovarian cancer and had plagued so much of

Maria's life – I could have given it to my daughter changed everything. Instantly. My grandma had been ravaged by the disease, and in the end she had given up fighting it. Now I was cradling my beautiful little girl, who could have it too. That was the moment I decided I'd been an idiot and needed to be tested.

The next few days in hospital were a blur of learning to breastfeed and bathe a newborn, changing nappies, soothing and bonding with our new addition, but when I got home and had unpacked, I rooted out the letter from the drawer and made the phone call to the Centre for Life.

I explained why I was calling and what Dad's results had shown, and the lady on the other end of the phone informed me my nearest test centre was Great Ormond Street Hospital. I took their first available appointment in May, four months away. In the intervening months I spent hours with our perfect little girl sleeping on me while I'd use my phone to google everything I could about the BRCA2 gene. Rather than reassure me, everything I read seemed to be about odds, chances, statistics, increased risks, and none of them seemed particularly favourable for me, let alone the beautiful baby girl lying on my chest.

While no figures exist on how many women in the UK have the BRCA gene, there are plenty of statistics out there about how it increases your risk of cancer to potentially catastrophic odds. The thought I could have passed the faulty BRCA2 gene on to Faith was bubbling away inside my mind constantly. Every time I'd uncurl her little fist while she fed I'd wonder if the gene was in the very fibre of her.

I didn't speak to anyone about it, though; I didn't want to worry Hugh with something we didn't know I definitely had, so for those four months I stressed a lot in silence, which, when combined with post-partum hormones, meant I spent a lot of time in tears.

On the outside, everything looked perfect. Hugh was delighted with our baby daughter, we were finally a family of three; Faith was thriving, and while I'd had some bumps along the road and had to stop breastfeeding after a few weeks, most of motherhood was amazing. Faith was the best baby, a great sleeper, amazing feeder, smiley and happy all the time and barely grumbled. But I was plagued with the nagging thought I could have given her something which had killed her great-grandmother. With every milestone she reached, it felt like there was a grey cloud hanging over both our heads.

I was worried for myself, I won't deny that. I'd read enough to know that testing positive was serious and that I would probably require some surgeries if I was a carrier, but I was petrified for Faith and wracked with guilt at what I could have unknowingly done.

I'd spend hours reading internet forums with women who had the gene. So many of them had made the brave and selfless decision not to have biological children and here I was with my baby daughter in my arms, having cavalierly decided to put a letter away in a drawer for months when I was pregnant with her.

In my googling, I came across pre-implantation genetic diagnosis, a process similar to IVF, where potential embryos are screened for the BRCA gene defect before they are implanted, which means parents can ensure a baby born without the mutation.

While I didn't know whether I had the BRCA2 mutation, I realised that if I'd been aware that I was at risk before I had fallen pregnant and had been able to get tested, if my result had been positive, we might have been able to have a baby without me passing it on.

I don't talk about problems until I have a solution, though, and I didn't have one for this. Besides, Hugh's an optimist, I knew he'd tell me not to worry or give it headspace until we knew for sure what we were contending with. As one of the sunniest men I know, it's always been hard to talk about anything negative with Hugh and while it's a trait I adore in him, sometimes – like then – I'd wish he were a little different. He hates being brought down by potential negativity, and he's able to flip a switch in his head and not think about it until he knows something is a definite negativity, but it wasn't quite so easy for me.

I knew if I raised my concerns and worries with him, or bombarded him with statistics, he'd tell me I was worrying for nothing and that there was no point even thinking about what might happen next, or what we should do if I had it until I knew for sure. Hugh's great at compartmentalising those things; I'm not.

It's difficult to describe what the potential of having the gene does to you. On one hand, you don't have cancer, you don't have a diagnosis or an illness, so there's no point in self-pity. You're 100 per cent healthy, with no problem at all. But on the other hand, you could have genes in your body that might cause cancer at any second; on a cellular level, the tiniest thing could happen that starts a chain reaction that could change every single thing in your life. You could be making a cup of tea when a cell changes and becomes cancerous, and that's a weird feeling to reconcile and something that's hard not to think about a lot. It kind of feels like when they discover those World War Two bombs when they're digging up roads – they've lain there for decades, not damaging anyone, but the slightest thing could change all of that and set in motion a series of events that could ruin lives.

While I didn't share my worries with Hugh, nor my mum at this stage because I couldn't bear to distress or worry them, Viv was tougher to crack so it seemed fair to use her as my sounding board while I awaited the appointment. I'd keyed her in after Faith had been born and we spent a lot of time together when I was on maternity leave. She was more than a best friend and Faith's godmother, she was part of the family.

I'd call her whenever I was worried and our conversations usually went the same way.

'Shell, I know you're panicking about it, but until the test and the results there's nothing you can do…'

'I know that, Viv, but what if I have it, what if I've passed it on to Faith?'

'You don't know you've got it and if you have then you're ahead of the game, imagine the numbers of people out there who've got it who don't even know they have it. You haven't got cancer, you're not sick, you might have a dodgy gene but, if you have, then you've found out at the right time before it's caused any damage, and you can take precautions to make sure it doesn't turn into cancer. Everything is in your favour if it turns out you have it, but you have to stop thinking about it until you know for sure…'

I always felt better after talking to Viv, but if she gave me that pep talk once in the four months I waited for the circled date on the calendar to arrive, she must have given it to me twenty times.

The morning of the appointment, I sat patiently with Faith in my arms in a waiting room at Great Ormond Street, the first children's hospital in the UK. I remember thinking I didn't want to be there with Faith. She was well, perfect, pure, she didn't even need to be in a hospital and yet it was my fault she was there. Looking around, I felt overwhelmed with emotion at the smells, the sounds and the worried-looking parents walking through the corridors. I was still a bit hormonal post partum and the pain and fear etched onto their faces as I made my way through the hospital to the genetic department was so desperately sad.

My mind started racing faster than I was comfortable with. I tried to think about what I'd do if the test turned out to be positive. Tried to imagine how I'd deal with it, what it meant for Faith, for Hugh, for me. What we'd have to do to minimise my risks and how we'd both live with the impossibility of not knowing whether Faith had it or not. My research had told me she couldn't be tested until she was eighteen, as there was no increased link to childhood cancers with the BRCA gene mutation and she needs to be old enough to make the decision about whether to be tested. So, with my baby in my arms, if the blood they were about to take proved I had it, we'd have another eighteen years' wait to see if I'd ruined Faith's life.

I don't like to think too many steps ahead, though, and the thought of all that was making me feel queasy, so I fixated on Faith's eyelashes as she slept, while I tried to block it all out, wait patiently and calm myself down.

'Take a hold of yourself, Michelle,' I whispered under my breath. 'You're just here for a blood test, so stop overreacting. It'll be over in a few minutes, no point in second-guessing what the results might mean when they won't be available for a few weeks.'

By the time I was called in, I'd calmed myself enough to have the blood taken and remember my manners to say thank you, and that was that. I was soon back in the fresh air of Great Ormond Street, leaflets in my hands and the doctor's words that the results would take around six weeks ringing in my ears.

In the month and a half after the blood test, with doubt raging, I'd spend days either convincing myself I didn't have the gene or googling everything I could about it. Viv would check in constantly to see how I was coping and while she was always positive about the whole thing, I struggled to feel the same way. One thing's for sure, though – not a day went by that I didn't think about it and not a night went by where it didn't haunt my sleep, and the last thing anyone needs with a six-month-old is interrupted sleep.

I wanted to talk to Dad about it, but every time he called and I mentioned I was waiting however many weeks still, he'd get tearful and start blaming himself, and then I'd have to counsel him rather than him counselling me. No matter how much I told him it wasn't his fault if he had passed it on, he refused to listen. He'd get himself so wound up that after a while it seemed safer not to mention it until I knew what we were looking at.

Sure enough around five and a half weeks after the blood test, I unfolded a letter inviting me to an appointment to get the results. Again, there was that word, 'invited'. It still seems odd to use it in that way, even now.

Instantly overthinking the words printed in front of me, I blinked back tears and tried to ignore an impending sense of doom.

'We recommend you bring somebody with you…'

It could have been a standard letter they used, just a

template that they added your name and details to, but what if it was the standard letter they sent out for people who have the faulty gene? I could feel my heart starting to pound, as I tried to reason with myself.

'Maybe it's the letter they send out for people who *don't* have it, so they'd have someone at the appointment to celebrate with, Michelle...'

I kept telling myself it could be that, because the other option seemed too unbearable to think about.

I showed Hugh the letter when he got home from work, but he didn't proffer an opinion either way, and while I knew he was trying to assuage my fears by not choosing either option, he can usually calm me down with a few words when I get upset, but not that night.

I spent the night not sleeping, holding Faith for way longer than I needed to on her night feed. It felt like I was on the brink of something huge – what, I didn't know, but I knew I wanted to savour the last few days of blissful ignorance before everything potentially changed forever.

Hugh was always going to come with me, but even with the letter and all my night-time musings, when we parked near Great Ormond Street that August, my swingometer of uncertainty had convinced me I didn't have it. Faith was just eight months old, and we took her with us.

Getting dressed that day, I honestly thought finding the gold heart pendant I wanted to pair with my orange vest was about the most taxing thing I'd have to contend with that day.

I'm not naïve and I'm no fool. I knew my great-grandmother, grandmother and father all had the gene, but I didn't think it'd be me. Three out of four was bad enough, it wouldn't be a clean sweep of a 100 per cent of us; it couldn't be, could it? I was well, healthy and had never had any unusual symptoms, surely that was a sign I was clear, wasn't it? Besides, I had heart problems from my arrhythmia, surely that was enough for me to contend with in life; I didn't need to add a hereditary cancer into the mix.

I'd spent eight months worrying, and the emotional pendulum in me had swung from being sure I had it to thinking I didn't. If the appointment had been a few weeks later, it probably would have swung the other way again, but on that day, if I'd been a gambling woman, I'd have put money on the fact I'd be BRCA2 negative.

We saw the same doctor who'd taken my blood test and when we walked in, she didn't make eye contact, instead busying herself with the papers pertaining to my test on her desk. I searched for her eyes but they were fixed elsewhere, while I felt mine fall away from hers and down to the floor.

I swallowed hard and I knew.

'There's no easy way to say it, you've tested positive for the BRCA2 mutation...' she said, raising her eyes to finally look at me.

I couldn't bring myself to look at Hugh as the doctor held my gaze. I felt my eyes well up and I wiped at them with one hand, clutching Faith tighter with the other while I searched her face for some morsel of news that meant it wasn't that bad, that I had a little bit of the gene, that she'd got it wrong, that it was some kind of new harmless type they'd identified just that week. But there was nothing.

I looked up at the ceiling, half to try and stop the tears falling and half to try and make sense of the words I'd heard. I desperately tried to swallow down the rising panic and quell the pounding sound of my heartbeat in my ears, but I couldn't silence any of the noise that felt like it was thundering in my chest.

Faith. My beautiful little girl, my perfect daughter.

She'd just weaned and learned to crawl. She loved playing peekaboo and could stack cups. She laughed easy and slept hard. My Faith.

If I had it – if the gene that would change my life had come down the last four generations – what was to stop it coming down a fifth? Jolting me back to reality, the doctor asked if I wanted to know anything about the genetics or if I needed them explained to me. I shrugged and looked to Hugh for the first time; his face was ashen, tears falling silently down his cheeks. We wouldn't walk past this, we couldn't. Negativity had hit us both right between the eyes, and now we'd have to deal with it.

He broke his gaze away from the floor to hold mine, both of us searching one another's faces for some way to make sense of it, some sign or fleeting glimpse between us which would signal it would all be OK – that we'd weather the storm we'd just unwittingly and unwillingly wandered into.

The storm we were completely unprepared for.

I felt awful for him instantly. He'd just been delivered the same bombshell I had, but he was helpless and could do nothing. I had the gene, he couldn't fix it or get me something that would make it go away.

And if I had it, his daughter could have it too.

My Menopause Musings

It took a nurse and having a baby to make me get tested for the BRCA gene mutation and for anyone who has living relatives who have had breast or ovarian cancer, it's a phone call and a few short questions to see if breast cancer or ovarian cancer is prevalent in your family. If it is, and your doctor believes there's a strong enough link, you'll be able to have genetic testing for free on the NHS. If you suspect you're at risk, make an appointment and speak to your GP.

If you've recently found out you have the BRCA gene mutation, you should have been offered genetic counselling. If not, ask your GP or genetic testing centre why not and follow it up.

Having the BRCA gene mutation is a very difficult issue to come to terms with. You have the potential for cancer, not cancer itself, and that's an uneasy bedfellow to get used to. If you're not careful, it can start to consume every thought and make you worry about every glass of wine or fast food meal you have, but that's no way to live. Do your research and find social media pages that can help you decide what path is best for you. I chose testing; when Dad finally got hold of David, he didn't want to be tested.

There are so many Facebook pages filled with amazing women, all on their own paths, with different advice and experiences. For me, immersing myself in it and reading as much as I could from women in the same situation helped inform the decisions I made. Some of the stories I read were from women who opted for watchful waiting and that worked for them; others had keyhole procedures on their ovaries, some the same mastectomy and reconstruction I had, but all of the stories I read were useful in informing me and helping me come to the decisions I did. Only by arming yourself with as much knowledge as possible will you be able to determine what will work for you and your family.

Of all the women I've spoken to, women who opted for all kinds of different paths and procedures, the one thing they all have in common is that they made the decisions that they felt were best for them.

Search Facebook for BRCA and you'll find hundreds of groups all across the world, filled with women all on the same journey at different times. The support you can get from complete strangers should never be underestimated. Reading other people's stories of strength and resilience bolstered me up many times as I navigated my new reality and helped me feel less alone when thoughts of BRCA and surgery kept me awake in the middle of long, lonely nights.

CHAPTER 3

The BRCA Bombshell Fallout and New Boobies

Hugh has the biggest heart of anyone I know. If he can make things better for me, he will in a heartbeat. Whether that's getting me a bottle of wine on the way home, even though he's teetotal, or whether that's training with me to make sure I stay motivated, he'll do anything to make my life easier, happier and healthier. But in that moment he couldn't do a thing.

The appointment where I found out I had the faulty BRCA2 gene lasted forty-five minutes, but in reality, my head wasn't in the room after the first three minutes. We were told there was up to an 85 per cent chance of me developing breast cancer and a 40 per cent chance of me developing ovarian cancer. Where the increased risk of breast cancer was concerned, she explained a preventative double mastectomy was an option, or watchful waiting, where I'd have regular mammograms, could be considered too. A hysterectomy that would put my body into surgical menopause in my thirties was an option to reduce the risk of ovarian cancer or, again, monitoring was an option.

It was too much, and I started to zone out.

I'd heard of mastectomies and I knew what hysterectomies

were. My mum had dealt with menopause in her fifties, so I knew what that was too, but I was in my thirties. I'd just had a baby, I was at the start of my fertility, not the end of it, surely?

Trying to make sense of what I'd heard so far meant I didn't listen to what else was said. I kept repeating what she'd said over and over in my head, and while I could pick out a few more words – 'cancer', 'breast', 'ovarian', 'aggressive', 'survival rates', 'surgery', '85 per cent likelihood' – the rest of it all went over my head. I was breathing hard, with Faith asleep on my lap, trying not to stir her while attempting to take in the hard fact that I'd have to undergo two operations, two big procedures.

On autopilot, I smiled and took every leaflet the doctor gave me, looked at them but didn't read any of their titles. I wasn't paying attention and I couldn't tell you a single full sentence she'd said. I nodded when she asked if I wanted to make an appointment with a genetic counsellor, but not a word came out of my mouth.

As soon as I heard there was an 85 per cent chance I'd develop breast cancer and that one of the options was a double mastectomy and reconstruction, I was planning it in my head. I'd been sideswiped by the results; in that meeting room, as my heart pounded and I collected leaflet after leaflet, I swore I wouldn't be unprepared on this journey ever again.

It's with the power of hindsight now, writing this, that I know I made the right decisions, regardless of how hard the outcomes have been. Simply being told I had the faulty gene shocked and floored me in that moment; the thought of what a cancer diagnosis would have done to me proves to me that I made the right choices, no matter how tough my experiences have been.

The doctor asked again if we had any questions, both of us shook our heads solemnly and she said a letter would come through the post for the genetic counselling appointment and another for a follow-up with another doctor, who'd discuss surgery options with me.

We meekly thanked her and walked out of the room in a daze.

Neither of us said a word until we were in Nando's. I ordered a huge glass of red wine and cried into it. I cried through my chicken, and while I told Hugh I wanted the surgery. I talked him through my plan for a double mastectomy and reconstruction and, having heard the increased risk that I'd develop breast cancer, he was right behind my decision.

'Whatever you want to do, however you want to go forward and whatever happens, I love you and I support you. I'm here and we'll make it through, OK, Shell?'

Before I got the chance to call anyone my phone rang. It was Dad, to ask about the results.

'Dad, please don't be upset. You don't need to apologise, I'm all right, I haven't got cancer.'

'I'm so sorry, Tuppence…'

I spent the rest of the conversation making sure he was OK. He felt so overwhelmingly responsible for what he'd passed on to me and what it'd mean for the rest of my life going forward. I always end up feeling guilty when I talk to Dad about it, purely because he feels so much guilt himself. Of course it wasn't his fault, it's never been his fault – it's genetics, and there's no blame. But he gets so upset at the thought of what he's done to his Tuppence, I have to assuage his tears before we can talk about what's going on with me.

'I'll be fine, Dad, don't worry. I'll deal with it and I'll be OK. I'm a lot better off than the thousands of people who received a cancer diagnosis today so don't panic. I've got to call Mum, so I'll talk to you later.'

One large swig of wine later, I called Mum. Like Dad, she'd been waiting by the phone for me to call once I had the results. She too had been sure I'd be OK and telling her wasn't any easier than telling Dad, although her reaction at least brought a smile to my face. Having come to terms with the devastating blow of Dad ending their marriage, she'd hardened her heart a little bit towards him.

'Your fucking father... Oh sweetheart, I'm so sorry, love, I really am, shall I come down? That fucking man...'

'It's fine, Mum, honestly, I'll be OK, it's not his fault.'

'Of course it's his fault, everything is his fucking fault...'

Mum and I are very similar – neither of us has a filter and we both say what we're thinking. That's why she's both my best friend and my most honest critic, we're like one person.

Despite having been on the phone for the first fifteen minutes of our meal, I'd been thinking while talking and had been multitasking, using Hugh's phone for Google searches while I talked on mine. I searched for what specifically would happen in a mastectomy, what would happen in a reconstruction, what kind of scars I would have, whether I'd be able to keep my own nipples, how long it'd take for the cells taken during the mastectomy to be tested for cancer or precancer, when we'd get the results of those tests, what the treatment options would be if the tests were positive.

As well as protein, that meal was about damage limitation, processing and preparing, so I wouldn't be caught out again. It was one of the most devastating pieces of news any woman could have received, but during that peri-peri chicken, I googled a plan of action, learning all about what procedures I'd have done. Applying logic to it all meant I was able to process it in pieces rather than let the whole of it consume me like an avalanche. Every time I thought of it all as a whole, it was too much. Tears would threaten and I'd have to swallow hard, but breaking it down into smaller, easier-to-cope-with chunks or steps meant I could think clearly and not be overwhelmed by the weight of it.

Having made the decision to have the surgery, the wheels were put in motion. The geneticist referred me on to a specialist breast surgeon, who would handle my mastectomy and reconstruction.

As I waited for appointments and surgical consultations, I was kept busy with everything I had going on and the rehearsals for *The Big Reunion*. It was going to be one of the biggest working periods of my life since Liberty X; we'd be rehearsing as one of thirteen bands getting back together, and filmed as part of a reality TV programme which would culminate in live shows and a tour.

I was beyond excited, I'd bought tickets for Five when I was a teenager and I'd be performing on the same stage as them. It should have been one of the most amazing times in my life, but I'd spend hours in between rehearsals and soundchecks researching everything I could find about BRCA.

It felt like I couldn't learn enough about it; the surgery and how long I'd be out of action, research into the gene, treatment breakthroughs, the history of it and when it'd first been identified and isolated. It was like I was revising for a test and I wanted to know everything off by heart.

One evening, two weeks before the surgery, I put Faith to bed and sat Hugh down after dinner for a talk. I'd tried to broach how I felt a few times but had always chickened out, or Faith had started fussing. I'd thought long and hard about what I was going to say and had rehearsed it in my head all day. I hoped I could get through it without tears, but sitting opposite Hugh, I could already feel them threatening to fall. I pursed my lips, took a deep breath and swallowed the tears back down.

'Hugh, I want to talk to you…'

'What about?'

I could already feel my voice starting to catch in my throat but I pushed on, regardless.

'I know I don't have cancer and I know everyone dies some time and that no one lives forever, but the reality of having this gene fault is that I'm at an increased risk of dying before I'm supposed to. I've never really thought about death, but it's a possibility for me because of this gene. It's a time bomb that could go off any second.'

'I know, Shell, that's why we're getting the surgery.'

He was looking at me with the big blue eyes I love with all my heart, and I could see him searching my face for some clue as to where I was going with it.

'Hugh, let me finish. If anything happens to me, I want you to find someone else.'

'Will you shut up?'

He went to stand and pick the plates up to take them into the kitchen; it was supposed to signify that the talk was over and he didn't want to hear where it was going, but I touched his wrist and implored him to sit back down again.

'Please, Hugh, listen and let me finish. You're such a good man, if anything were to happen to me, I'd want someone to experience what a good man you are. I can't picture you growing old or Faith growing up without a female figure in your lives.'

He could see that tears were streaming down my face and he moved to sit on the bench next to me, holding my hands in his as he did.

'Michelle, nothing is going to happen to you and even if you walked out on me tomorrow, I never want anyone else. I only want you, I love you and we're going to grow old and grey together, OK?'

I fell sobbing into his arms and held him the tightest I ever have. My rock. We were looking into a storm but holding Hugh then, I cried like I hadn't since getting the results. While I was terrified of what the storm might bring, having my husband beside me made me feel brave enough to weather whatever it threw at us.

I had an elective double mastectomy and reconstruction in November 2012. After a five-hour procedure and recovery, I groggily awoke to a heavily bandaged chest. I'd lost my breasts and reduced my risk of developing breast cancer. I was floored when I came round. I couldn't say a word. Hugh kissed me on the forehead and cheek while I tried to bring my faculties into focus again. I didn't realise, but he'd been holding my hand while he'd waited for the anaesthetic to wear off.

Piece by piece it came hazily back; I'd had the surgery. I was in hospital. My risk of aggressive breast cancer had decreased from 85 per cent to hopefully around 3 per cent, if the breast tissue they'd taken was all clear.

I looked down and, beneath the heavy bandaging, I could make out the shape of my new boobs; they didn't seem so different to what I'd spent the last thirty-three years looking down at.

Hugh caught my gaze and smiled, then gently reminded me that a team from the *Lorraine* weekday morning show was waiting to get a few words from me after the operation. I can't specifically recall the moment I decided to go public with my diagnosis and my decision to have this procedure, but I think it was mostly because I hated the thought that people would think I'd had a boob job – the reconstruction I'd opted for post mastectomy – for vanity.

Not that I have any issues at all with women who do that – some of my very best friends have had several enhancing procedures, because they can and because they want them – but it just didn't seem right in that instance, for me, that people would think I'd done it for fun. I was doing it to potentially save my life and the only way to let people know that was to talk openly about the journey I was on.

Lorraine Kelly has a strong track record in covering issues that matter to women; I'd been on her show before and liked the team and the nurturing environment the show is made in. I had spoken to them about following my progress through surgery and recovery, and they immediately decided they wanted to.

Hugh told me they had spent the whole day at the hospital. I found a clock on the wall of the recovery room and calculated they'd been there roughly fourteen hours, a long day by anyone's standards. They didn't need much, but I'd known going under the anaesthetic they needed something. It had seemed fine then but post-operatively, I had no idea how I felt.

I could feel myself starting to cry. 'Hugh, just tell me what to say. I don't know what to say...' I trailed off as he wiped the tears from my eyes.

'Tell them it's all over. Tell them we can move on and it's all done, then they can go home and you can get some sleep.'

I motioned towards the door and minutes later the camera was rolling.

'It's all done, a weight's been lifted, the cloud's gone. I can just get on with life now.'

They backed out and left the room. I was exhausted.

I was in hospital for five days; Hugh came every day with Faith. I missed them both dreadfully and while I felt lighter at the prospect of having reduced my risk of breast cancer, I mourned for the old, complete me.

When the nurses took the dressings off and unravelled me, my new boobs were very swollen and it looked like I'd had a big boob job done and gone up several sizes, when I'd actually stayed the same size. They looked vulgar and I didn't like them at all. I tried not to panic, though, and focused on context. I'd reduced the risk. That was what was important.

Vivianna was a regular visitor too and would tease me, telling me my new boobs were much nicer than my old ones. I loved her visits because she always brought a smile to my face. I had a drain in each breast, which hurt every time I moved, despite the high dose of tramadol, so laughing wasn't actually what the doctor ordered.

With time in hospital, I did everything I could to reconcile what had happened, to come to terms with it all, but to this day it's still hard to explain how I felt or how that operation changed me forever, mentally as well as physically.

Each woman will answer differently if you ask her to tell you what makes her a woman, what makes her feel feminine. With potentially lifesaving surgery to focus on, I hadn't dwelled too much on how much my femininity would be affected by the mastectomy and reconstruction, but I felt less of a woman as I recovered during those first few days in hospital. My old boobs had felt part of what made me a woman. The implants didn't have the same emotional attachment.

On the one hand, I'd had a treatment which would keep me alive for longer and, on the other, I'd had a procedure some women use to boost their self-esteem. The two elements didn't sit easily together.

When I got home, Mum came down from Gateshead to look after Faith while I recovered. The minute she came through the door, I asked her if she wanted to see them. I knew her face wouldn't lie, couldn't lie, so I knew showing her would help me gauge whether they looked OK or whether they looked hideous.

I've always been close to Mum, but I'm not sure I'd ever flashed at her before, but before she'd even had the chance to take her coat off, I showed her the results of the reconstruction.

'Oh, Michelle, they look great. They look so normal and you don't look like you'll have much scarring, pet. You must be delighted?'

'They don't feel like mine, Mum, they feel weird and I haven't got much sensation in them.'

Showing Mum my new boobs didn't feel like I was showing her my boobs, it's why I'm fine to show them (after a few wines) to women who are considering the procedure themselves. I'd never have shown anyone my old boobs, my real boobs. But these are fake, they're not real, they're pretend and they're not mine, so I don't feel protective or embarrassed at showing them. For me, it feels like I'm showing a thing rather than a part of me. My physical recovery was textbook, and Hugh's definitely a fan of how they look – so much so I fell pregnant with AJ a year later. Hugh and I had talked about having two children and while we hadn't been trying, we both knew we didn't have all the time in the world.

We knew there was a risk I'd pass on the gene, something we hadn't had to consider with Faith because we didn't know back then, but we didn't have the chance to talk about it at length for a couple of reasons; firstly, while AJ was planned in the grand scheme of things, he wasn't planned specifically and so falling pregnant with him was a surprise, and secondly, I was still adjusting to what the gene meant for me and learning all about BRCA. If the developments I'd learned about and the pace of discovery and change I'd read about was anything to go by there was a huge potential that a child born in the noughties with BRCA would face a very different future to a child born in the seventies and diagnosed with BRCA. I suppose we both hoped the medical landscape would be a completely different one by the time any child we had who might have the gene grew up and the risks of what the gene could do became real.

My risk of ovarian cancer increased every year I went further into my thirties. A geneticist at Great Ormond Street had told me that the age at which the BRCA2 gene mutation stopped being dormant often ran in families, ergo because my grandma had it around my age, it was likely that if I was to develop it, I'd have it in my thirties too.

A hysterectomy had been mooted when I'd had my mastectomy – a two-for-one kind of operation where I'd have both procedures done in one longer surgery, rather than undergo two general anaesthetics and two recoveries. I could have opted to get it all done in one go, but Hugh and I knew we wanted to expand our brood and give Faith a sibling. Both of us had grown up with siblings, me with my brother David and Hugh with a sister. We knew how much that dynamic had meant to both of us. With a 40 per cent risk, we felt it worth waiting an extra year or so and so we'd precariously hedged our bets.

We'd had conversations about the fact that the gene would ultimately lead to me having a hysterectomy and we knew that was what we were looking at once our family was complete. We'd decided before we got married we'd stop our family at two, and so with AJ growing safe in my soon-to-be-removed uterus, I made an appointment with my specialist to discuss options for the operation.

With ovarian cancer the biggest risk to me, there were options of just removing my ovaries (an oophorectomy) or going the whole nine yards and getting rid of everything (where they would remove my womb, fallopian tubes and ovaries). I decided to opt for the latter.

While my obstetric gynaecologist, Mr Sheridan, might not be everyone's cup of tea, he certainly was mine. He was the specialist who'd delivered Faith and, because I trusted him so much, he'd deliver AJ and then six months later he'd perform the hysterectomy. Anyone who's dealt with him will have an opinion on what he's like; when I went to my ten-week scan, he told me – without asking if I wanted to know – that we were having a boy.

'But, Mr Sheridan, you didn't even ask me if I wanted to know the sex and Hugh isn't even here.'

'You didn't find out with Faith and everyone always finds out with the second baby. Besides, Hugh won't mind not being here, I know what he's like and so do you.' He was right, I knew Hugh wouldn't be bothered that I'd found out ahead of him and I'd been intending to find out at the seventeen-week scan anyway. 'If it's not a boy, I'll eat the placenta. Now hurry up, I've got other patients to see and I'll see you in a few weeks.'

While I feigned annoyance, his straight-talking, shoot-from-the-hip attitude appealed to me massively, which is why he was the man for the job of my hysterectomy. I didn't want to be hand-held through it, I wanted someone who'd be honest and tell me the facts of what I was looking at, and Mr Richard Sheridan most definitely is that man.

It felt bizarre having conversations about AJ and the hysterectomy at the same time, but the weeks and months were ticking on. After I'd recovered from having AJ and was able to dedicate some time to him, I'd go back into hospital again for the hysterectomy which would plunge me into menopause.

While I knew I'd have the hysterectomy, I had different options of keyhole or abdominal surgery, and Mr Sheridan helped me decide which to have. He explained in his usual matter-of-fact way that, having had a caesarean section with Faith and another one planned for AJ, anatomically, things might not be where they expected them to be – that in closing me up after two caesarean sections, things could have moved around a bit.

Removing my ovaries would be a keyhole procedure and I'd be up and about the same day, but there was a chance they'd try to locate them and they wouldn't be where they should be. In which case, while I was under they'd have to convert from keyhole surgery to full-on abdominal surgery. Basically, I'd go under anaesthetic not knowing whether I was looking at a few days' recovery or upwards of months.

With my job unpredictable at the best of times and with no family living nearby to help out, it wasn't a risk we could take. I always need to know my schedule for work and I have jobs booked in up to twelve months in advance. The way Mr Sheridan suggested it – leaving it to chance on the day – just wouldn't work, professionally speaking. The other option was to have the hysterectomy at the same time as the caesarean section but that seemed too immediate.

For some reason, the thought of going into hospital pregnant with a baby growing in my belly and coming out of hospital with the very organs that had sustained life gone forever – it didn't sit well with either me or Hugh, like we'd be getting rid of something too soon. After long talks between us both, we scheduled the surgical hysterectomy for six months after AJ was born.

My Menopause Musings

I've been exceptionally lucky that I have a document of a time in my life that was incredibly difficult and traumatic. Having the *Lorraine* team there to film my mastectomy made a huge difference to how I looked back on it and remembered it. So much so, I continued making videos of my recovery when I got home, to document it for us all, as the children grow up and as it all fades from memory.

If you're not comfortable with videos, take loads of pictures of the procedures you go through on this journey, whether it's pictures of you mid-hot flush, or immediately after a hysterectomy. Whatever you do, pictures are a really visceral reminder of how far you've come.

Rewatching videos of me after the mastectomy shows me how much I've improved, how my confidence levels returned gradually, how I recovered. I took videos of myself pregnant with AJ and I'd video my thoughts and musings when I came out of appointments with Mr Sheridan. They're not all for public consumption and I look pretty dreadful and groggy in a lot of them, but they're for the children when they grow up and I'm glad I bothered to do them.

CHAPTER 4

My Baby Boy, Meningitis and Las Vegas

Aaron Jay Hanley came into the world on 28 February 2014. He was 6lb 5oz.

After a few minutes of post-birth tranquillity, my newborn son, AJ, moved his little head and the peaceful skin-on-skin contact which was bonding us turned into a gentle nuzzle and then a rooting.

A panic washed down from my head to my stomach as my beautiful son, my darling AJ, tried to nuzzle for sustenance that wouldn't come. For food I couldn't give him. My naked breast, which had been gently rising and falling with every breath, started to heave deeper, tears beginning to swim in front of my eyes.

The nurse who'd helped him into the world continued watching with a smile, sure that any second he'd find the nipple, latch on, start feeding and she'd once again witness a bond from birth between a mother and child.

Hugh saw the first tear trickle diagonally from the side of my eye towards my jaw. Our eyes met and I saw pity flit across his face. He opened his mouth and looked towards the nurse.

'I can't feed,' I whispered, as much to my son as to the nurse.

'It'll take a little bit, but you'll get the hang of it,' she replied, not understanding what I said, not hearing the grief of the admission I'd made.

'No, I can't feed him because I've had a double mastectomy,' I explained, the tears streaming harder.

While she took a second to register and understand, AJ knew instantly and his murmurs turned into wails of discontent. In the space of a few seconds, all the euphoria I'd felt on his arrival dissipated. Replaced by guilt, with failure echoing close behind.

There was no milk.

I couldn't nourish my son.

My attempt to prolong my life through preventative surgery meant I couldn't give AJ what he needed the most. What he needed to survive. Emotionally vulnerable, physically exposed, our two bodies wracked with sobs, our bond switched to emotional and actual hunger; Hugh cried silent tears too, and the nurse excused herself to go and find a bottle and some formula to silence and sate my sobbing son.

In that moment, something broke in my heart and my head. Looking down at the baby I'd grown and cherished, I wanted to undo everything. Undo the feelings of guilt which felt overwhelming, undo the first time I'd ever heard 'breast is best', undo the double mastectomy so I could feed AJ the same as I'd done for his sister, undo what felt like a widening chasm between us.

In the few minutes as I waited for the nurse to return, the noise in my head desperately tried to reconcile what had happened, to put it into some kind of greater context and not let the feelings of failure and guilt take root. I tried to push against the first swells of postnatal depression that rose higher and stronger with every single one of his tiny, hungry cries.

It doesn't seem to make much sense, but in the nine months I'd been pregnant, I hadn't considered the fact I couldn't feed him. Faith had taken a day or so to start feeding and I'd put her onto bottles within a few weeks of her birth. With a full hysterectomy scheduled months after AJ's birth, rehearsals for a new tour, Faith to nurture and a family and work to juggle, I hadn't factored formula or bottles into the bag I'd packed for the hospital.

It simply hadn't occurred to me at all.

I felt I'd failed as a mother on so many counts. What kind of a mummy can't feed her son? What kind of a mother doesn't think about it ahead of time? His first minutes should have been filled with love, tranquillity and happiness, and instead they'd been filled with sobs, hunger and a gut-wrenching sadness, which felt like it was breaking my heart.

I could see Hugh's tears as we both waited for the nurse to return; I was able to silence AJs cries with a bottle but mine continued to flow. I was defeated and while I smiled down at my newborn son, as he greedily sucked on a rubber teat, gulping down what I couldn't give him, I felt a rift develop between us. I loved him and I'd failed him, just minutes into his beautiful little life.

Those feelings of having failed him took months to abate; I was an emotional wreck post partum and would cry every time he cried. The guilt felt enormous, which is why it felt both flattering and emotional when I had a call when he was two weeks old, telling me I'd been chosen as the Disney Celebrity Mum of the Year. I'd known I was in the running before having AJ, but up against Davina McCall, Coleen Rooney and Danielle Lloyd, I'd told myself I didn't stand a chance. Both

Faith and AJ were supposed to come with me, but Faith had been sick in the car on the way and Vivianna, who was helping me out by coming too, decided to take them both back to hers while I concentrated on work.

I spent the entire day answering questions about motherhood and how incredible it was to win, all the while still feeling like I'd failed AJ. I spoke about the fact I couldn't breastfeed him because of the mastectomy and reconstruction, but I didn't utter a word about how emotional that had made me and how all over the place I felt about failing him. I put on a brave face and pretended everything was perfect. The irony of being voted Mum of the Year when I was about to have all my 'mum-making' organs removed wasn't lost on me either. Here I was, being celebrated for motherhood just months before that option would be removed forever.

It was a strange day and while the award is exceptionally flattering, it came at a hugely emotionally volatile time for me. A time that also wasn't helped by the fact my beautiful little boy battled meningitis at six weeks old, which was utterly terrifying. As he lay in a hospital bed, I blamed myself again, wondering whether his immune system had let him down because I hadn't breastfed him. I was supposed to be a Mum of the Year, yet all I felt was failure.

It was without a doubt one of the worst times of my entire life, but being the tough little fighter with the gentle heart that he is, after being touch and go for a while, he pulled through and grew strong enough to come home again.

Having had Faith in 2012, a mastectomy the same year, AJ in 2014 and then spending weeks in hospital with him at six weeks old, battling a potentially fatal virus, when Hugh suggested we take a week's holiday in Las Vegas with friends before I had my hysterectomy, I jumped at the chance. It'd been a tough few years and while our amazing little family felt complete, we had one more huge hurdle to get over, and it felt like the biggest of all.

While my recoveries so far had been OK, even when I got better from the physical surgery of the hysterectomy, I would be going into surgical menopause and neither of us had any idea what the fallout from that would entail, how long it would last or how easy it would be to adjust to. With a gruelling few years behind us and a tough couple of years ahead of us, we decided to take a minute to celebrate what we'd been through and to steel ourselves for the next battle. This was a 'life is about to change forever' holiday. AJ was six months old and – each to their own – we felt we could leave the kids without it being a big deal, so Mum came down to look after them.

I'd had two years of stress, worry, anxiety, operations and sleepless nights, either with the babies or BRCA2. Hugh could see I was emotionally exhausted and running on empty and with a holiday on the horizon, I did what I always do when I'm worried or stressed and have an event I want to look good for… I hit the gym. I'd work out early, determined to be shredded for poolside cocktails in Vegas. I'd gained 3st during my pregnancy with AJ and, while the hysterectomy date was circled in red on the calendar, I focused more on the Nevadan sunshine than what would happen a few days after we returned.

We both looked forward to what we knew would be an amazing holiday, some much-needed 'us' time away from everything we'd had to contend with in the last couple of years. It'd be like we'd be able to press pause on all the stress for a brief moment. Knowing I had the faulty BRCA gene was still something that made me emotional and while I'd removed – literally – my increased risk of breast cancer, the fact I still had my ovaries meant I was constantly living with a higher-than-average risk of ovarian cancer. Having that hanging over me was completely exhausting.

Vegas seemed such a decadent choice too, so filled with lights, noise, life and fun; it felt like the perfect tonic for a pair of sleep-deprived parents of two kids under three. It was incredible. Our first and only time away from the children, and a chance to be Hugh and Michelle again, not just Mummy and Daddy. The penultimate day, while we were beside the pool in thirty-degree heat, sipping iced tea, Hugh interrupted my dozing.

'Shell, are you OK about next week?'

'What do you mean, Hughie?'

(I know I'm the only person in his world who calls him that.)

'You know, the operation. Are you feeling OK about it?'

'It is what it is…'

I tailed off and pretended to be snoozing, but the reality was I'd tried not to give it too much thought. I so wanted to enjoy the holiday, I'd locked the prospect of my third huge abdominal surgery in three years safely away in a box marked 'do not open' in my head. I was physically over the mastectomy, I'd had AJ and got back in shape; being returned to thoughts about BRCA2 felt like a step back to a place I wanted to forget.

I'd spent the week watching beautiful women around the pools and casinos of Las Vegas, and while there were lots of fake boobs on display, I reckoned they all still had their female organs intact. They were all-woman and I was about to undergo a procedure that would remove all the internal organs that I felt made me a woman. I was willingly getting rid of what made me hormonally and anatomically a woman. All the women I saw that week looked like they'd be able to carry a child, and in a few short days that option for me would be gone forever.

Looking down at my abs, I felt like in a week's time I'd be just a body. Not a woman, a body. The Michelle who had given birth to two beautiful babies would soon be just a shell, unable to ever do that again.

I'd spent hours in the gym, training so I looked good in Las Vegas, and every time the procedure had popped into my head, either during a workout or while I was with the kids, I'd pushed it firmly to one side and tried to replace it with thoughts about our holiday and sunshine and time spent with my husband, or I'd do another ten reps, so all I thought about was the workout. I didn't want to think about it, I didn't want to accept it. I knew enough – or so I thought – to go through with it and that was that. I'd figure the rest out afterwards.

Besides, what very limited research I had done on the surgery – reading leaflets I'd been given – told me millions of women across the world have the procedure every year and they all seemed to recover, if not thrive; I'd work my way through it just like every other woman seemed to. I'd read stories of women on social media groups talking about their experiences and while they hadn't always been positive, I honestly didn't think all that much about the harder, longer recoveries some of them had described. I'd reckoned that being in my thirties would stand me in good stead, that my journey wouldn't be as tough, or my recovery as arduous, as some of theirs had seemed. I was young and fit, surely I'd be fine?

Snapping my thoughts back to the warmth of the day, before I started getting overwhelmed by anxiety about the operation and my recovery, I reached over and squeezed Hugh's hand.

'Don't let the operation shade the last day of the holiday, Hughie, we'll talk about it when we get back. What do you want for lunch? I'll go and order something.'

While he tried to hold my gaze to see what I was really thinking, I closed my eyes again in the sunshine, waiting for him to answer. He took the signal as it was intended, that I didn't want to talk about it or answer any more questions about it, and, thankfully, he let it lie.

My Menopause Musings

Finding out I had the faulty BRCA2 gene and then having the mastectomy and reconstruction soon after felt necessary for me, but it wasn't an easy surgery to have. I know and respect many women who have had mastectomies and opted not to have reconstruction, but it was the right thing for me to do at the time.

Friends would tell me how amazing my new boobs looked, but getting used to them wasn't easy. I hadn't been unhappy with them in the first place and the fact I'd had no choice (as far as I was concerned) to get rid of them meant I took a while to settle into my new breasts (more of that later).

While I opted to have the reconstruction done at the same time, I was also given the option of a mastectomy and then a reconstruction further down the line, something a lot of women I know have chosen to do and have been completely satisfied and happy with.

What I do know about the first surgery is that I couldn't have gone through with it without the support of friends and especially family. Hugh was a rock through it all and I'll never be able to thank him enough. He knew just when to order me some tempura and sit beside me in pyjamas watching a DVD and when to get me into my gym gear and out for a workout. While I'm not prepared to share him with anyone just yet, if you're on a journey like this or something similar, find your rock and let them help you through.

There were so many times I thought twice about telling Hugh trivial little things about my experiences and the surgery and the gene but, through sharing everything, he got to walk a little in my shoes and, because of that, he was able to know when I needed sympathy and calories and when I needed sweat and a workout.

I know not everyone's lucky enough to have a significant other, so whoever you have in your life – parents, siblings, online friends – there's no need to go through anything alone. If you need support, you can find it; but in order for that support to really make a difference, you have to be open too.

CHAPTER 5

Surgery Setbacks, Hair Thinning and Binge Eating

When we got home, we didn't pick the conversation up where we left off in Vegas. Hugh didn't ask the question again when we landed on home soil and in the ten days between landing at Heathrow and driving to the hospital, we didn't speak about the emotional upheaval we were about to face, we just talked practically about the impending operation. We talked about juggling the kids, Hugh's work and the time he'd have to take off; everything that would logistically affect our lives and jobs, but nothing that would emotionally affect our marriage. We had no idea at all what we were about to walk into, in that respect.

In the fallout that followed the surgery I tried – as I always do – to put on a brave face for Hugh, or at least not panic him as much as I was panicking myself. What good would sharing the fact I felt like I was falling apart at the seams have done? It's not that I was keeping anything from him, but sharing it seemed pointless. He couldn't fix it and neither could I.

Although I'd been advised to rest for at least a fortnight, I'd booked work into the diary, not anticipating how much the procedure would take out of me. After the operation, I'd already started to worry about work, but Hugh had made his feelings clear – he thought I needed to reschedule and move some commitments, but I'd refused, initially thinking I'd feel better day by day and be ready to resume a workload exactly when I'd said I would.

While my recovery felt completely different to what I'd expected, I awoke every morning in the hopes that whatever day it was would be the one, the game-changer; that I'd feel less like an old woman, broken inside and out, and more like the woman who'd gone in for the procedure, the woman who had enjoyed the sunshine of Las Vegas just a few days before.

The reality, though, was very different.

Slowly lowering myself into the car four days after the surgery, Hugh looked down at me, his face fraught with worry.

'Shell, are you sure you're making the right decision?'

'Hughie, I'll recover much better at home. The doctors have said I'm on track, if they were adamantly against me discharging myself I'd listen, but they're not. I hate the food in hospital and I hate sitting watching the clock, waiting for you to come and see me. I hate the smell and the sheets and everything about it. I'll take it easy at home, I promise, and I know I'll recover faster with you, Faith and AJ around me.'

Missing the kids had been the biggest part of my desire to come home but in all honesty, the carb fest I was being fed every breakfast, lunch and dinner was starting to make me feel bloated and sick. Even Vivianna was sick of jacket potatoes, and that's saying something.

I longed for my regular diet of plenty of vegetables, lean meats and healthy light meals. In hospital, every time I'd move, my bloated abdomen would weigh heavy and feel disgusting – like it had a mind of its own. At least I'd be in charge of what went into it if I went home, and I figured that would help both my mental state and my physical recovery at the same time.

The first day or so at home, I stayed true to my word and spent most of the hours on the sofa resting, sleeping and finally eating better. Faith would cuddle up next to me, we'd read together or watch cartoons. Hugh would bring me AJ to feed and cuddle too. But by the end of day two, my trips to the toilet – until then my only time spent vertical – started to include trips upstairs to pick up some toys in Faith's room, or trips to the kitchen to put some dishes in the dishwasher, or some clothes in the washing machine.

Whenever Hugh caught me, he'd get cross and shepherd me back to the sofa, but sitting and lying down all day didn't agree with me. I hated it. Recovery was boring. I wanted to be recovered.

Mum came to help with the children when Hugh went back to work, but she'd come downstairs from having played with them in their room to find I'd made lunch for us all. She'd shout at me and tell me I should be resting, but I resented all the time I was spending on the sofa and wanted some kind of physical normality back, even if the emotional one was nowhere to be seen.

Despite Hugh's protestations – and he made many – ten days after the operation I stuck to a commitment to film a live segment for the *Lorraine* show. I'd fronted their Bin Your Bra campaign for breast cancer awareness month the previous year and they'd invited me back. I'd accepted the job before the surgery and had figured ten days after it I'd be able to get back to work – if not in the full swing of it then at least almost back to normal.

I couldn't have been more wrong. With staples still in my

stomach, the feeling of carrying a huge weight on my back and the inability to stand up straight for more than a few minutes at a time before becoming the Hunchback of Watford, I presented three days' worth of live feeds from different Tesco's stores across the country.

The producer for the show – who spent the days ashen-faced with worry – would have a chair just out of shot, and the minute the segment would finish she'd push it behind me so I could gently lower myself onto it and rest in between feeds back to the studio.

I was presenting live and learning my lines, all while in a near-constant, head-spinning level of pain. I shouldn't have even been standing up for more than a few minutes at a time, let alone standing in heels, pretending nothing had happened. I was loaded up with pain medication to try and get through the job, and the pencil skirt I wore would send a shooting pain through my scar every time I moved.

In between shots, I'd switch from heels into flats because I couldn't stand. I'd sit until they started a countdown and then said 'go', and then I'd stand and do it again before sitting back down. The pain medication I was on gave me mouth dryness as a side effect, so with the nerves and the medication, I felt like I was barely intelligible.

After every day, Hugh would pick me up and I'd move towards the car at a snail's pace, completely exhausted and utterly spent. The second I'd climb in, the professional mask would slip and I'd sob in pain the whole journey home. I'd collapse onto the sofa or bed when I'd get in, and Hugh would have to bring me something to eat before I'd fall into a fitful sleep. Every move in the night would send pain searing through my abdomen and then every morning I'd do it all over again.

But the reaction to the campaign was amazing. So many women got behind it, and the social media feedback I had personally really bolstered my flagging spirits daily. The incredible women I spoke to and the response the campaign received made that job one of the hardest yet one of the best of both my BRCA2 gene journey and of my working life so far. The campaign raised millions, the hashtag trended and women from all over the country got in touch with me to tell me what they were doing to fundraise for such a vital cause.

A few days after filming *Lorraine*, I had my staples removed. Mr Sheridan was happy with my recovery so far and how it was progressing – I decided not to tell him I'd already started working again. He said I'd need some more post-operative outpatient appointments to make sure things were still going to plan, but so far so good: my recovery at that point was what he expected.

It wouldn't stay that way, though.

The same day the staples came out, I decided to try a little stroll out with Mum. I live about half a mile away from a Costco, and it seemed the perfect little jaunt out – we'd get stuff done and take it easy. AJ was in his buggy and while Mum offered to push him there, I was adamant I could do it.

I could feel it starting to hurt before we were through the first aisle. Seeing the pained expression on my face, Mum went to take the buggy and push my son for me.

'I'm fine, Mum, honestly, don't worry.'

'Michelle, I'm not worried, but you look like it's sore, why don't you let me push him?

'It's OK, maybe in a bit.'

By the time we sat down in the canteen for hot dogs and pizza, my abdomen was hurting even more.

'Michelle, why do you push me away, why don't you let me help? I'm here to make things easier, but I can't do that unless you let me.'

She was right, as usual.

'Sorry, Mum, I should have, but I hate feeling like I can't do things myself. It's so frustrating. I should be able to push a buggy.'

'And you will be able to, you've proved you can, but don't do it to the detriment of your recovery. Don't let that stubborn character you get from me slow you down. Take the help and recover properly, OK?'

'OK, thanks, Mum. Can you push AJ home for me?'

Reaching over the table and squeezing my hand, Mum stood, planting a kiss on my head and taking charge of AJ.

She was right about my stubborn nature, and it'd rear its head again a few days later.

While Mum gave me the character that won't accept help easily, both my parents gave me a Northern work ethic. It's ingrained so deep in me; I stuck to another commitment to present at the Baby Show at London's Olympia exhibition centre less than two weeks after the operation and just a few days after I'd had the staples removed from my stomach. The added pressure involved in this job was that when I'd agreed to present, I'd also agreed to perform a workout from my pregnancy fitness DVD.

Hugh begged me to reconsider, but I refused.

The Baby Show is one of the biggest gatherings of pregnant women of its kind in the UK. I'd been booked months in advance; not going wasn't an option, no matter how I was feeling.

'Michelle, you're not well enough to perform a bloody workout. You have to cancel, you'll put your recovery back. Jesus, you only just had your staples removed, Mr Sheridan would go mad if he knew you were even considering doing this.'

'Hughie, I can't cancel, I've committed, and besides there'll be two models doing the workout, I'll only have to join in for a bit, I have to talk more than I have to move. Please stop worrying, I promise I'll be fine and I'll take it easy.'

The day of the Baby Show arrived and while deep down I knew I was in no condition to go, let alone perform a workout, I got dressed, loaded up on painkillers and stuck to the script.

An hour into what would be a twelve-hour day, I knew I'd made a huge mistake, but I didn't want to say anything because I had a job to do. A whole team of people, including the organisers and PRs for the show, were counting on me to do the workout and the talk. Sure enough, by the time I went on stage, the assembled crowd was one of the biggest of the entire day.

Anyone who was there that day will attest to the lacklustre performance of the workout – I did as much as I could without falling over on stage and left most of it to the models, but before the music even came on, I knew Hugh had been right and that I'd made the wrong decision. I got through it, but by the time I got home I almost fell through the door and spent the rest of the night in tears. I was exhausted, I felt close to breaking point emotionally and my abdomen was even more swollen than it had been post-operatively.

I'd known almost immediately that I should have gone home and I knew no one would blame me for backing out just a few weeks after major surgery, but my pride and my work ethic stopped me. I'd had plenty of chances to tell the organisers, who could have made small changes to what I'd do on stage, but I'd been stubborn and hadn't wanted to let anyone down.

I knew Hugh was angry with me, having warned me it was too much, and yet he made me a bed on the sofa and got the kids sorted while I slept. The minute I lay down I must have fallen straight to sleep because when I came round, it was dark and I couldn't hear the kids – a sure sign they were already in bed. As my eyes adjusted to the familiarity of the lounge, Hugh's worried face came into focus. He was searching my face for an expression which would tell him how I felt. I smiled and I felt him relax a little.

'Shell, you can't keep on, you've got to take care of yourself. You have to cancel some commitments and take your recovery seriously, anything could have happened today... We need you, you can't put yourself at risk like that. You could have opened the wound again, ended up in hospital, anything could have happened, which could have resulted in more surgery or more time in hospital...'

As he trailed off, I could feel tears pricking at my eyes. He was right. I'd been an idiot. Professional pride had been more important to me than my health. What was the point of undergoing these lifesaving procedures if I was going to put myself at risk post-operatively? I was going through all of this to be there for my family, so what was the point of risking short- or long-term setbacks?

The following morning, I made an emergency appointment with Mr Sheridan; after examining me, he told me I'd put my recovery back a fortnight because I'd tried to do too much too soon. I was crushed but promised myself, Mr Sheridan and Hugh I'd take it easy and listen more to my body.

Not only had I almost gone back to the drawing board, but my steadfast refusal to compromise my work schedule had meant instead of cancelling just one or two bookings at the start of my recovery, I'd have to cancel more in the coming weeks as I finally listened to my doctor's advice and properly rested. Worse still, because I'd done the workout at the Baby Show, one side of my scar had stretched and I'd left myself with a flap of skin on that side that would never go.

Over the next few weeks, as I allowed my body to begin its recovery properly, my mind started to unravel. I'd finally taken the doctor's advice about my physical well-being but my mental well-being was getting worse, not better. Although I knew counselling was available, and I'd been told I could book a session as an outpatient whenever I might decide I wanted it, I would have had to go and request it, and I'm not the type of person to ask for help. I should have done really, with hindsight, but at the time I didn't and that's not something I'm proud of.

Hugh was back at work and playing catch-up for the extra time he'd had to take off when my recovery was set back. He'd leave the house early and get back around 7 p.m., so it'd be 8 p.m. by the time the kids were in bed. Then, after dinner and a clean-up, we'd barely have an hour or two a day where we could talk. I didn't want to sound like a broken record, talking about myself all the time. 'How are you feeling, are you OK?' were the first two questions Hugh asked every day when he came through the door, but with the kids around and after a long day for him, there never seemed the right time to really

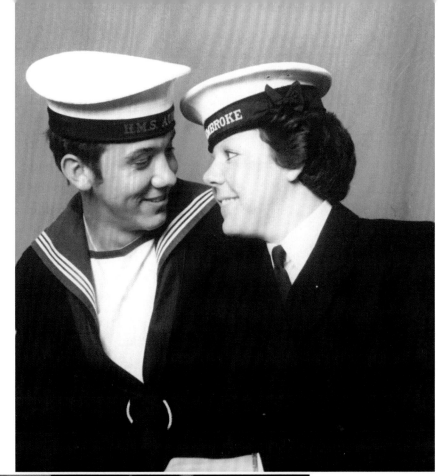

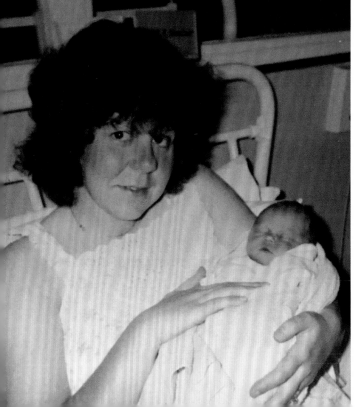

Above: My mum and dad – Christine and Chris – in their early twenties, both just about to leave the Navy.

Left: Welcome to the world, Michelle! I'm only a few hours old in this shot, taken on 19 July 1979.

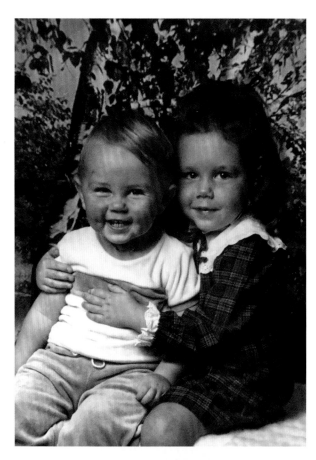

Left: With my little brother, David, in 1983.

Below: After winning a talent competition at Haven Holidays.

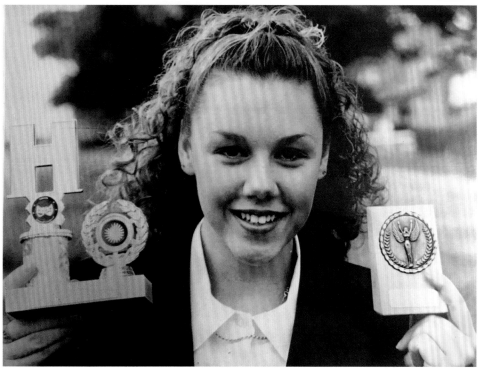

Right: Another award from Haven, this time in a regional talent competition in 1993.

Below: With my grandmother Maria in summer 2001. Maria had battled with cancer so many times, she was a real heroine to me.

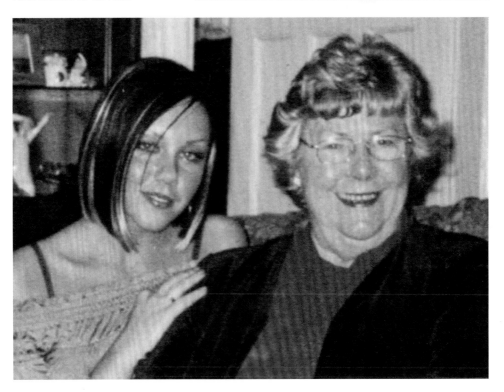

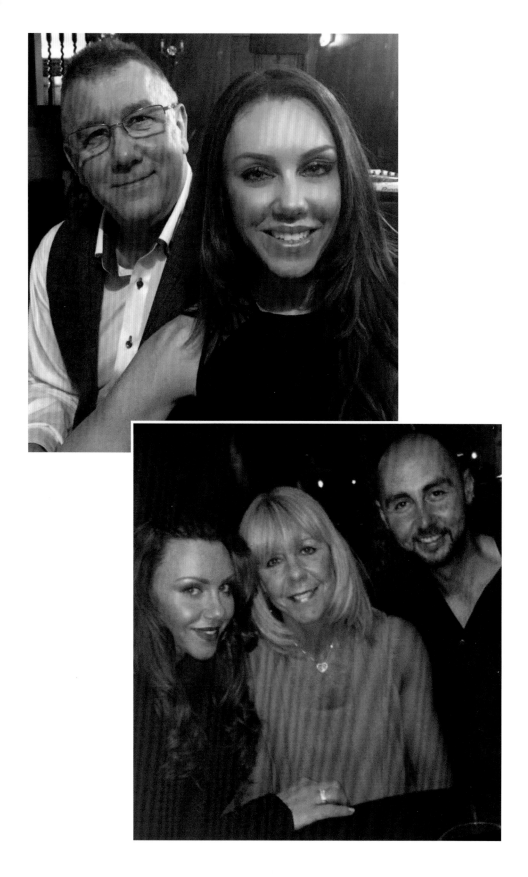

Top left: With my dad, who always called me by the nickname Tuppence.

Bottom left: With my mum and my brother David, before he left for his travels, summer 2011.

Below: With Hugh on our wedding day in the Bahamas, 19 July 2010.

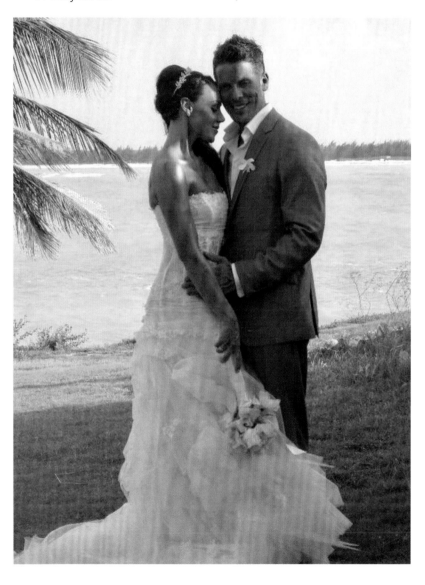

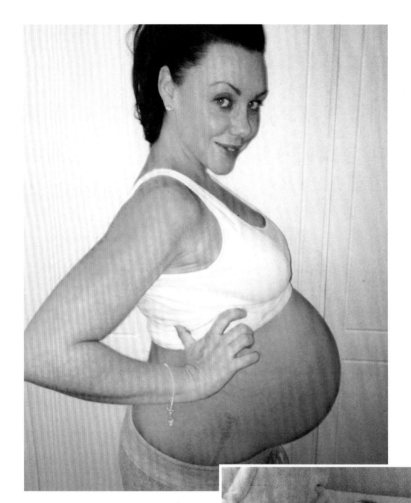

Above: Proud of my bump!
It was around this time,
pregnant with Faith, that I
decided not to get BRCA
tested and put the letter
away in the drawer.

Right: My beautiful Faith
was born on 11 January
2012.

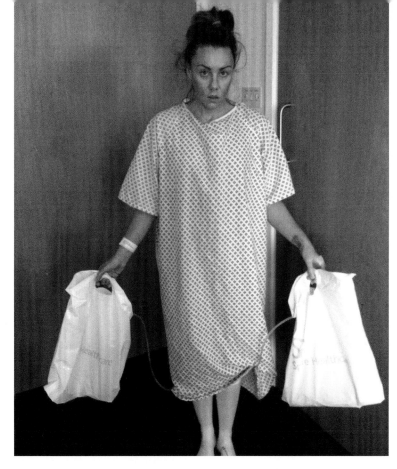

Above: Two days after the double mastectomy, with the fluid drains still in my breasts, November 2012.

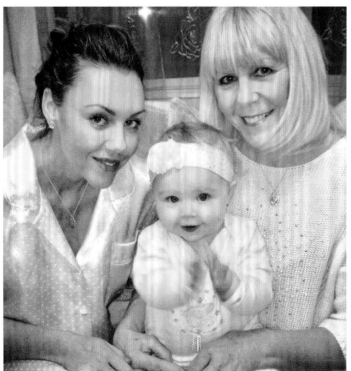

Left: With my mum and Faith, a few days after my double mastectomy, when mum came to help out at home.

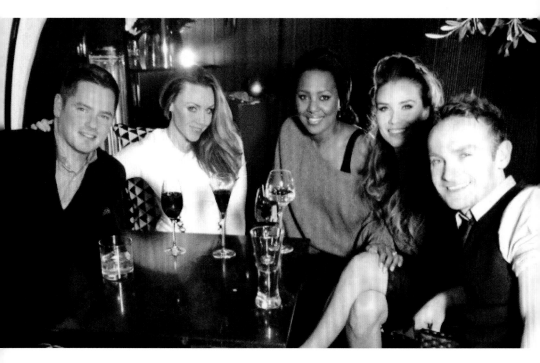

Above: Just a few weeks after my operation Liberty X had a big reunion, all meeting up again after a five-year break.

Below: These shots were taken just before AJ's birth in February 2014. Faith couldn't wait for the new arrival and kept reassuring me that everything was going to be OK.

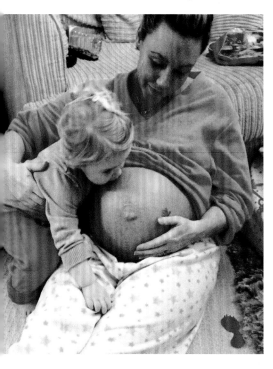

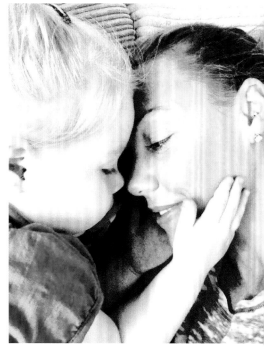

be honest and tell him how I felt. I spent weeks hoping that as my body recovered, my emotions would somehow right themselves too, that I wouldn't spend all my time seconds from tears or feeling angry and upset. I'd never felt emotions on such a swingometer before and they were exhausting. I didn't want to talk to Hugh because I didn't understand them – and I wanted to, before I shared them. I had no idea what was going on myself, so explaining it to anyone else would have been near impossible.

Vivianna and my mum were always there at the end of the phone, but again, I struggled to explain how I felt; I couldn't put my finger on it enough for it to make sense, so while we spoke almost daily, I didn't talk about the growing feeling that I was falling apart emotionally. I couldn't share it with Mum because she'd already been upset, telling me she felt useless, that she couldn't do anything to help or make it easier. I couldn't talk to Dad because he'd have become emotional and upset, blaming himself for my situation, and I didn't want to have to parent him through his guilt. So I did what I'd started to do more and more: I kept my feelings to myself, tried my best to understand it and spent my recovery trying to deal with it on my own. I didn't and don't want people to feel sorry for me, but I felt like I had no one to talk to. No one to help me come to terms with it all.

Having been knocked sideways by the emotional fallout immediately after the operation, I was now having to try and process the longer-term emotional and physical effects of my body adjusting to having every single natural hormone ripped out and synthetic ones put in. During the surgery, Mr Sheridan had inserted an implant that would slow-release my first dose of HRT and reduce the most significant symptoms of menopause. He'd made clear the dosage would need to be adjusted as my body and hormone balance altered after the operation, but initially I'd just have oestrogen implanted. He explained they could change the dosages and prescription every six months, but with hormones being unlike any other medication, the effects wouldn't be instant and so it could take a while to hit on the prescription that would work best for me going forwards.

I spent a lot of time thinking about womanhood and what it meant after my surgery – whether I still felt part of that group. In the absence of the internal organs that made me a woman, I began to focus on external signs that would anchor me as female; looking as feminine as possible suddenly became one of the most important parts of my recovery. It became increasingly necessary to me to make sure my hair was done and my make-up perfect. I booked several appointments to make sure my nails were always freshly done. I couldn't control how I'd been cut open, stitched up and put back together, but controlling my external appearance became, and still is, a huge priority for me. Whether I'm in the minority, the majority or somewhere in the middle, I don't know. I know anecdotally from the women who message me and contact me on social media that a lot of women in menopause and women who've undergone hysterectomies feel the same.

The ability to have children – whether you want to or not – is something every woman I know feels strongly about. Now, not only could I not have children any more, but I didn't have my own boobs either. As I gingerly started doing more, I'd find myself trying to reconcile myself to the contradiction I felt – I outwardly looked female but nothing inside me suggested I was still a woman, or at least that's how it seemed. I had pretend boobs and pretend hormones, no ovaries or womb, and I couldn't adjust to life with all of that gone and everything fake. I didn't feel like me; everything which had once been mine was no longer in me, replaced instead with synthetic materials.

While innocuous-looking letters have dropped onto my doormat in the past and blown my world apart, a year or so after the hysterectomy I received a letter that played right into the anxieties I have about feeling like a woman and being a woman. It was from my local hospital; they were writing to advise me I wouldn't be invited for cervical screening any more – so far, so fine, I didn't have a cervix any more, after all.

But their wording hit a nerve of insecurity which did little but compound the tumultuous feelings I was wrestling with about not having womanly organs any more. I read and reread the letter until I'd almost learned it word for word.

Dear Mrs M. Heaton,

We have been advised that your name should be removed from the list of women eligible for cervical screening. This is because your medical records indicate that you do not have, or no longer have, a cervix. I am therefore writing to confirm that you will no longer receive invitations to screening.

If you believe this information is incorrect and you should still be called for screening, please contact this office as soon as possible.

It felt so inhuman, so unfeeling, that it was hard not to feel upset and angry. A simple human sentiment like 'I'm sorry to hear that' would have made it so much better to read. I couldn't help but feel a growing sense of anger about the impersonal nature of it. It was so detached, whereas it was discussing something incredibly emotionally charged for me. How could someone have approved a letter like that going out to women who don't have a cervix, for whatever reason?

I took to social media, posting the letter on Instagram. I didn't do it to shame the NHS that I love so much, but simply to gauge whether my reactions were in line with everyone else's thinking, or whether I was overreacting because I was so sensitive about the whole subject. The response I got was staggering. Women who'd had the same surgery as me called for the hospital to apologise, others suggested I lodge a formal complaint and lots of women told me they'd received exactly the same letter. Whoever devised the draft hadn't even considered the effect the wording would have and with my emotional state on the whole femininity issue wobbly before I got the letter, it made it a whole lot worse.

During one of my musing periods a couple of months after the operation, while Faith and I shopped at the supermarket, I felt a gentle tap on my shoulder.

'Excuse me, I'm sorry to bother you, you're Michelle, aren't you?'

'Yes, hi, how are you?'

So far, so normal. I'm usually stopped a few times a week and Faith didn't bat an eyelid, accustomed to strangers talking to Mummy. I always try and be courteous and kind because nine times out of ten people just want a chat.

'I just wanted to say because of you, I got tested for the BRCA gene. I saw you on *Lorraine* and have followed your story ever since. I found out six months ago I have it and I've just had a double mastectomy and hysterectomy too. I'd never have been tested for the gene if it hadn't been for you, so I wanted to say thank you. You could have saved my life.'

'Oh my goodness...'

I swallowed the lump in my throat as she continued.

'You've been so brave, and seeing how you've coped with it has given me strength. You're an inspiration, and I've really appreciated your honesty. It's definitely helped me. Seeing what you went through gave me permission to feel low and down about it.'

We talked for a few minutes about how we both came to the decision to have hysterectomies and mastectomies – like me, she was a mum, and while we were both dealing with an emotional and physical fallout, knowing we'd be there for our children longer was the kernel of hope which we both pinned our decisions and recoveries on. We talked about how it felt, potentially passing that on to our children, and while I'd never laid eyes on her before, we had so much more than just a gene in common.

When she said goodbye, the tears I'd kept in check came spilling out. Faith squeezed my hand.

'Mummy, can we get some yoghurt? Did that lady make you sad?'

I crouched down to her eye level, hugging her into me and smelling her strawberry shampoo. 'No darling, she's had the same tummy problems that Mummy's had. She's had an operation too, to make her all better and she's got children like you and AJ, who she loves just the same way I love you...'

'Oh, I love you too, Mummy, what's for dinner?'

In the coming weeks and months, I had thousands of messages: letters to my agent, tweets, social media mentions, emails and people stopping me in the street. They told me that seeing what I went through gives them permission to feel how they're feeling, or that they thought they were alone with a symptom or an emotional fallout until they saw that I'd felt it too.

Knowing that someone else is going through it or seeing that they're in pain never gets any easier to deal with. I can see so much of my journey in their faces and seeing them as lost as I felt is always difficult, not least because I can't help. It also reminds me of how rudderless I felt after the hysterectomy when I first entered surgical menopause.

I always listen and I'm always honest about my experiences so far and how I came to decisions and how I reconciled it all. I can't say what they're going to experience because everyone is different and no two BRCA gene journeys or menopauses are the same. All I can do is tell them what's in this book, in the hopes that they can prepare more and weather the storm a little better than I did at the beginning. I don't want to say anything that will make people make the wrong decision; I'm only meeting people for a few minutes of their life, I can't tell them everything in those few minutes, especially if I'm with my kids or they're with theirs.

They don't know it, but their honesty and their comments always give me strength too, despite the fact we might be at completely different points in the road. Sometimes speaking to a woman who's just been told she has the faulty gene reminds me of how far I've come since that diagnosis, since that room at Great Ormond Street Hospital, since that Nando's meal when my world felt like it was caving in.

I don't see myself as others do, I don't think my decisions have been inspirational; I don't think I've been brave, I haven't done anything spectacular or amazing. I've just made decisions as best I can, based on what life has handed me. It wasn't bravery; I couldn't have continued living with breasts and ovaries that could have potentially killed me. I'm not unusual in that.

The women who stop me in the street, or at an event, or on the way to the supermarket are the ones who are behind the decision for me to use my voice to speak out about menopause and the BRCA gene. Their stories and their bravery and bewilderment make me want to carry on doing what I'm doing and trying in a small way to raise the profile of the journey I and every single other woman in the UK will end up on. Whatever vehicle comes to me to keep talking about menopause, I'll take, because I know what a difference it makes to the women going through it. Some were yet to make the decision after finding out they had the BRCA gene mutation, some were getting tested because of family histories. Even men stopped me, telling me their wives had found my story useful.

Not everyone who stops me has the BRCA gene; hundreds of women who I speak to every year are going through menopause for a variety of reasons, and they're always grateful to me for trying to bring it out of the shadows. In those first few months after the hysterectomy, despite feeling like I was adrift and struggling in my recovery, if the people contacting me were anything to go by, I was helping hundreds of women.

While my physical recovery continued and I was back in the gym, training again – albeit gently – my emotional recovery was becoming increasingly difficult to manage. In addition to trying to assimilate the Michelle I'd thought I was before going under anaesthetic to the one who woke up, my reflection added to that growing sense of unease and change that – try as I might – I couldn't shake off. I hadn't felt like me when I woke up and while I was still wrestling with that and trying to get myself back to some kind of normal, my reflection looked nothing like the 'me' who had gone to Vegas or gone to the hospital for a hysterectomy.

Within months of the operation I started to notice my hair thinning. I first noticed it when I was tying my hair back at the gym, and I realised I was able to loop my hairband round my ponytail an extra time, but I didn't think too much of it to begin with. But then my hairdresser, Inanch, who is based on Great Portland Street in London, mentioned it to me. I've been to her for the last ten years, and she knows my hair better than anyone. (In an industry that values thick tresses, it's something I stress about a lot still. It's uncomfortable to go out and not feel my best, but that's what I have to do every day because of it. I don't know if or when it might stop thinning – it's a result of the imbalance in my body of oestrogen and progesterone. Without hair extensions, my hair snaps and breaks, and while I know I have to take breaks from them occasionally, I hate it when I have to; my self-esteem plummets every time.)

And while the initial swelling of my abdomen began to go down a little, I was still having to take it easy months after the operation – which frustrated me no end – and the body which I'd been getting back into shape after AJ seemed a million miles away at that time. This was not helped when I look at my incredibly ripped husband, whose job is all about fitness.

Hugh's never judged me physically and he never, ever would, but he's always inspired me to be the best version of myself that I can be, so the fact I was nowhere near that version of myself really messed with the low confidence levels I'd experienced since the day I came round from my surgery.

It's also no secret I struggled with an addiction to diet pills in the noughties, so it's safe to assume my self-image isn't the most positive or centred it could be all the time. Add in the fact I work in an industry which judges on the physical, a smattering of the hard truth there's always someone younger coming through in the business and the certainty that unless I'm seen out and about, looking great, the work won't come, and I had myself a recipe for some severe self-loathing and panic about my reflection.

I built my career in a period of the British press where no holds were barred. I was constantly labelled as 'the fat one' of Liberty X and considering the fact I was in my early twenties when I joined the band and had come from a council estate in Gateshead, that level of critique had a massive impact on me. I don't get criticised any more because the media knows what's happened to me health-wise, but it's had a lasting effect on how I view myself. I'm far more critical than any journalist in the early noughties could be.

Cue binge eating.

Since the operation, I'm still waiting to look at my reflection and really, truly like what's looking back at me, and while I've battled food demons in the past, I have an issue with food now I didn't have before I went into menopause, and I think that issue was sparked in part by how ill-prepared I was for the physical changes that greeted me.

The feeding and bingeing tendencies that I go through now – are they hormone-related, are they control issues from the reflection that greeted me when I woke up? Does every woman have the same issue in menopause? I don't know, but from the women who I speak to, I'm in a minority but by no means alone.

I do know the hormones ghrelin and leptin are the ones that control appetite and I know they can vary and change during menopause. I do know research from Oregon Health and Science University found monkeys with diminishing levels of progesterone and oestrogen increased their food intake by up to 67 per cent, and I do know I have to tackle the bingeing tendencies that started post-operatively and still happen now, because they're contributing to a lower confidence level which I'm trying so hard to build up.

When I binge, it's not just a little bit either. It's a lot and it can go on for days. A few months after the hysterectomy, Hugh and I went to Gilgamesh, in Camden, London. We'd arranged it as a night out, just the two of us – which happens really rarely. Hugh knew I needed some time with him and having already started making sure I always looked as good as possible after my hysterectomy, it was a nice excuse to get dressed up and have some much-needed 'us' time.

The menu is exquisite; so much beautiful food, sublime sushi, to-die-for tempura, delicious dim sum. We had an incredible night and while we touched briefly on how I was feeling, it was an amazing evening, which gave us a glimpse of what we'd been like before the hysterectomy. I finished the meal thinking things were getting better, that the old life I'd enjoyed could come back and that I was just recovering still. Hugh was full to bursting and we enjoyed all the food we could eat – or at least he did.

On the way home, though, despite having had more to eat than my husband, I still wanted to eat a petrol station cheese and onion sandwich and salt and vinegar Discos. We argued about my greed until he gave up and pulled into a BP on the way home, and I got my way.

'Michelle, you can't still be hungry! What are you doing? How have you got room?' He turned it into a joke about my appetite being bigger than his, but that's a classic example of a bingeing episode – when one hits, I have zero self-control.

While we joke about it if Hugh's present when a binge happens, he'll never understand why I overeat to the point of sickness. My relationship with food has a long and turbulent history, and the fact my metabolism has slowed since menopause – a natural side effect – means the weight is easier to gain now and harder to shift, which has deepened my sense of self-loathing.

It's a pattern of behaviour that I didn't have pre-menopause and the bingeing can happen for days on end.

I don't know if it's about control, punishment, both or neither. What I do know is that it's a cycle; I eat dirty and gain weight, then my reflection confirms physically how I feel emotionally about myself and gives me the justification to loathe myself. Then I eat more because I'm down.

I can fluctuate by at least two dress sizes between a Monday and a Friday, from a size 8 to a size 12, and that's not something that I ever did before the operation. Being 5ft 4, that's a big swing in weight and a fair few inches round my waist too. I've never talked about it before for plenty of reasons and I'm not asking for sympathy, just a little empathy. Even at my heaviest during a binge, as a size 12, I know I'm still fairly slim by other people's standards, it's just that I'm not by mine and while I'd never tell anyone else how to feel about themselves, I hope some of you can understand where I'm coming from.

When I get to a point where I know I've gained weight in a week and the scales and my skin confirm it, there's a switch that happens in my head and I'm able to drag myself back onto the wagon but then I'll punish myself in the gym. I'll work twice as hard as normal, do a juice detox for a few days and drink gallons of water, and I'll lose it and get back to normal.

I know it's not healthy and because I'm only admitting it here for the first time, I've not sought help for it before. It's something that's not completely in my control, but I do know it never spirals to the point that I spend weeks bingeing and continuing to climb up the scales. There's a tipping point for me every time I binge: a pair of jeans that when they get tight, I know I need to do something and get myself back on the wagon.

I've never spoken to Hugh about it, but being my petrol station chauffeur, he can see I'm bingeing and he knows I don't have the healthiest relationship with food. I don't know why it's been exacerbated since the hysterectomy, but I do know the bingeing cycles I'm constantly prone to now are somehow very deeply ingrained into my menopause journey.

My Menopause Musings

One of the biggest things I wish I could have changed about those early days, weeks and months post-op would be permission I refused myself. I didn't give myself permission for anything: to feel low, to cry, to rest, to binge, to self-loathe, to find it hard.

I felt guilty for not cleaning and tidying the house, I felt guilty for not working harder, working better, working longer, being slimmer, bouncing back. I felt guilty for not being as emotionally resilient as I had been before the operation and I didn't once give myself a break or even entertain the idea that it could all be related to the operation and procedure I'd been through.

I didn't give myself permission to struggle, which is why being stopped in the street and told I was an inspiration just made me tearful.

I'm gentler on myself now than I was after the operation, but it took me a long time to accept things weren't going to be how I thought they were, both immediately and in the months and years since I went under the anaesthetic.

Menopause is tough enough without constantly thinking and feeling I should be coping better, or should be working harder, or cleaning more, or being a better mum, or a slimmer me or a happier me.

I still have negative cycles, where I binge and I'm hard on myself and I hate my reflection – seeing only the bad parts of it. But every time the negative cycles strike, I try and remind myself I'm alive, I've reduced my risks of cancer and that should be the focus, the benchmark against which I measure all other emotions.

Whatever stage you're at, giving your feelings permission to exist will make them easier to deal with in the long term, even if they're negative feelings and even it doesn't feel like that now. You're not supposed to bounce back, you're not supposed to pick up where you left off, it's OK to not like yourself for a while, to be confused, upset, to act in a way you didn't before menopause… The sooner you realise all that and give your emotions a space to exist, the healthier recovery you'll have.

It doesn't mean you have to be happy with your feelings either. If you're having a fat day or you're not back on your feet as quickly as you thought you would be, it's OK to feel down and frustrated about that; no one's expected to love the feelings that come post-operatively but accepting they're as much a part of the recovery as the physical aspects will mean your road to recovery will be much quicker than mine.

CHAPTER 6

I'm Not Old: Fun, Anxiety, Friendships and Finding a Level

Anyone who's gone or is going through menopause with a young family will know children, no matter their age, wait for no one when it comes to their needs. It doesn't matter how little sleep I've had or how stressed or emotional I feel, the alarm goes off every day and Faith and AJ's needs take precedence over whatever I'm feeling or how I'm coping or not coping.

Fourteen months after the operation, my little Faith, growing bigger and feistier by the week, decreed that she wanted a proper birthday party with friends rather than family for her fourth year on earth.

She wanted cake, she wanted it at home and she wanted her friends.

She was in Beech class at her little school, and I asked her teacher to point out and name some children who she played with in the playground who might want to come. I had no idea sending out those invites would be the biggest change in my life and my friendship circle since my own school days.

The mums and their little ones all attended and because the

children were all only four, the parents stayed for the whole party, rather than leaving and returning at the end to collect them.

Faith had an amazing day, and I had one that helped my recovery more than I could ever have imagined – which will come as a surprise to them all reading this. Thanks to Faith and her four-year-old demands, I've made six of the most amazing friends I'll ever make. They've been pillars of strength for me in the last few years and – while I've never told them in as many words – they've been an integral part of my recovery and my adjustment to living with the menopause.

We have a night out every few months, which could be to the local pub or somewhere further afield, but it's always easy and it's always just us. We're all so different, too – no one else is in my industry or has the experiences I've had. There are stay-at-home mums, business owners, teachers, creatives; no two of us are the same and maybe on paper we shouldn't work as a friendship group, but the fact our children sought one another out as friends is a real anchor for all of us and maybe goes to show that four-year-olds are better at choosing their friends than some grown-ups are. Faith picked out some lifelong friends for me, and I'll always be grateful to her little demands for that.

I get to treat them occasionally too. None of them are in the media and none of them get the offers that I do, so where I used to drag Hugh along to things (sometimes under protest), now I have a friendship group ready and willing to take up opportunities and come with me.

It's not that they're my make-do therapists and it's not that I unburden to them or spend hours talking about what I'm going through; they're just an amazing group of women who provide fantastically hilarious distractions in an environment where I feel safe, loved and nurtured. I've been lucky enough to have made some amazing friends during my career who are in the same industry as me, they know who they are and they know how much they mean to me. But the Beeches Mums, as we christened our WhatsApp group, are a group away from that and I found them at a time when I needed close-knit, close-proximity friendships like that.

I don't meet the Beeches Mums at a posh London restaurant, having all spent ages getting ready and waiting to be photographed; I meet them on the school run when I'm exhausted and haven't slept and am in my gym gear. I'm not 'Michelle going through menopause' to them. I'm just Michelle, Faith's mum. They provide a safety net away from Hugh, away from my family and – like all safety nets – I hope I'll never need it, but knowing it's there makes me feel braver and more able to cope.

Hugh has to love me, it's his job, but these mums don't need to be near me, they're all busy enough with their own lives and jobs and children. The fact they choose to be and the fact they want to spend time with me has given me a confidence boost at a time in my life when I'd started to wonder whether it was a steady slope down from one HRT implant to another.

And it's not just the Beeches Mums who've been part of the wider circle of friends who've helped me through. I met Rochelle at a gymnastics club for kids when Faith was two, and she has become a lifelong friend and someone I've leaned on a lot. Rochelle's auntie had breast cancer, and it's prevalent in her family, which has meant we both feel incredibly strongly about the disease and how it can ruin lives.

But while Hugh has borne the brunt of some of my emotional fallout in menopause, it's incredibly hard to admit my friends have too – from Rochelle to Vivianna to the Beeches Mums, there've been times where we've argued and those arguments haven't been brought about by anger, like they are with Hugh; every single one of them has been because of an anxiety I have now, which I didn't have before.

A few months after the hysterectomy, I had a job in London to go to, and Rochelle had offered to come and sit with AJ while I took Faith with me. With timings tight and my fixation with never, ever being late, I'd spent the week texting Rochelle to remind her of timings. I knew she knew it was important and I knew she'd do everything she could to be on time, and she didn't have a track record for being late – in fact, she's one of the most punctual people I know. But I was nervous about the meeting and because I couldn't control the outcome of that, the anxiety I felt about it manifested as panic and a desperate urge to control everything else, from Rochelle's route to my house to her time-keeping.

Unfortunately, because of a motorway closure, she was late, which meant I missed my train, which made me late. There was nothing she could do, it was an unforeseen event and no one's fault at all.

Did I take it all in my stride? Did I text her and tell her it didn't matter?

No, I texted a barrage of upset at her, telling her it had ruined the job I might have been able to get and that she'd let me down. I was upset more than angry, and my text was blunt. Pressing send, I started crying at the helplessness of the situation and how awful I felt.

I know being on time is an obsession of mine and I know

– especially since the menopause – I'm not as good at dealing with things when they don't stick to the strict timeline I've set them. Rochelle couldn't help it, nothing could be helped, but I simply couldn't cope with the situation. I was helpless and because there was nothing I could do to undo what had happened, anxiety got the better of me and I hurt the feelings of one of my dearest friends along the way.

I called the person I was supposed to be meeting when the tears subsided and rearranged the meeting so I could take AJ with me. Once on the train, I texted her a huge apology. 'I'm so sorry I took my traffic frustrations out on you, it proves I feel comfortable with you but it also proves I'm a prat xxx'

I ordered her some flowers to be delivered the next day, but it wasn't until a few weeks later that I told her everything about the levels of anxiety I felt. I told her how I cannot cope emotionally if something goes wrong and I'm not able to control it. I explained how panic starts rising the second something doesn't go to plan and the old Michelle who could deal with panic can't cope so well any more. I told her about the vulnerability I feel when something happens that I can't fix. I told her about the times where every ounce of calm leaves me and I become physically tense, emotionally weak and anxious about everything. Rochelle being Rochelle, she was her usual kind and understanding self; she's always pretty calm and when I explained it to her with complete honesty, she tried her best to understand how it might feel.

When Vivianna has to cancel a meal we've had in the calendar for a while, I can't cope like I used to and I take it to heart. I would have brushed it off a few years ago, but I'm not as resilient now and I get really upset. Rather than see the cancellation for what it is – a friend rescheduling because she's busy – I start to wonder whether she still wants me as a friend, whether the fact I'm not the person I used to be means we don't have as much in common any more.

Family are supposed to support you come what may, but friends are about choosing, and why would anyone want a friend who drowns in anxiety the second something doesn't go to plan or a friend who questions herself and whether she's worth something the second a night out gets cancelled?

My friends have had to bear the brunt of my anxiety a lot over the last few years, and I'm grateful to them all for sticking around. My friendship groups have changed, evolved and developed in menopause and while things have adjusted and I've struggled at times, without the friends I have, I wouldn't be where I am. Their unending support, love and compassion has helped so much.

From long walks with Rochelle while I considered the decisions involved in my BRCA journey, to nights out with Vivianna where we'd spend hours talking about our old flat and nights out in Rotherhithe, to the Beeches Mums and after-school glasses of wine, my friends are some of the most amazing women and have been amazing to me.

But while they've been integral to my recovery, my inclusion in their lives and my need of them in mine has taken its toll on my marriage and it's something I'm still trying to balance. Hugh loves them all as much as I do, but with old friends and new ones to fit into an already busy schedule, there's even less time for my husband every week.

I get together with the Beeches Mums as a group at least once a month and I see them individually around once a week. I see old friends like Vivianna and Rochelle as often as I can too, and the fact that I have to be out in the evening for work once or twice a week – there's not much time left for Hugh and me. What time there is that is left for us, I'm either hungover or exhausted from work nights out or Beeches' or friends' nights out.

It's not that Hugh has dropped to the bottom of my priority list, far from it, but the amount of quality time we're spending together has decreased. Especially since the Beeches Mums became part of my life, Hugh's grown increasingly worried about the amount of time I'm spending out and the amount I'm drinking when I do go out. They're the new addition to an already packed schedule and he's worried they could be the straw that breaks the camel's back.

Is he justified? Maybe.

Do I like it when he mentions it? No.

Am I out far too many nights a week for a married woman? Yes.

A few months after meeting them, while I was getting ready for a night down the pub with them, Hugh sat on the bed as I put my make-up on.

I know him better than he knows himself and so paused, turning to face him, waiting to hear whatever it was he needed to get off his chest.

'Shell, you're socially active a lot of the time, I feel like I'm not seeing you. And don't take this the wrong way, but you're drinking a lot too…'

'Hugh…'

'Hang on, let me finish. I don't mind the drinking and I think it's just as a consequence of the fact you're out a lot, but I want to check you're OK, that there's nothing we need to deal with? You've incredible self-control, I know that, but I'm worried about you. I miss you and while I know this friendship group means the world to you, I love you too…'

Tears brimming in my freshly mascaraed eyes, I sat next to him on the bed, hugging him close. He'd said something out loud I'd been thinking inside. I knew I was going out a lot, Hugh and I were still adjusting to life post hysterectomy and neither of us knew which way the chips were going to fall when they eventually did.

I was still incredibly emotional and volatile, and my moods were nowhere near the level they're kind of returning to now. Things were up in the air, and I think my husband was worried he was losing me to nights out or a better or different alternative. The words came tumbling out as I looked at the ceiling, trying not to completely wreck my make-up.

'Hughie, we're married, you'll always be the top priority in my heart, but I know you've been the bottom priority in my life for a while and I'm sorry. That's not been on purpose, I'm just trying to keep every plate spinning. You work full-time so I have the kids all day; I need to be out at least twice a week to keep work coming in and to make sure I'm on people's lists for campaigns; the Beeches Mums are a real lifeline for me, and I don't want to start leaving my old friends out in favour of my new friends. I know I've been drinking more lately and I've noticed it's too much, too, but I'm not dropping any balls. The kids are fine, I'm still working out, the house is still clean…'

I trailed off as I searched for some kind of resolution, something I could say which would make it better. Hugh took the opportunity to talk.

'I know you're busy and I know you try so hard to keep everyone happy, but you're the only one I care about and I want *you* to be happy. If you're having fun and enjoying yourself that's fine by me, but if you're stretching yourself too thin, you'll snap at some point and you've been through so much already, I don't want that to happen to you...'

While I'm often the ringleader with the Beeches Mums, suggesting the extra bottle or that we switch to spirits as the end of the night approaches, that night I made my excuses and came home early to my husband, my rock, my world.

My Menopause Musings

I learned from my Beeches Mums, friends and my conversations with Hugh that everyone needs a recipe for what works for them in menopause.

It's such an uncertain and unpredictable time. Your emotions change hourly and that's exhausting in itself. Not to mention the fact you'll never, ever know what reactions and behaviours are really, truly you and what reactions and behaviours are because your emotions are in free fall and you might not have the right cocktail of HRT sorted yet.

After much sampling and too much of one thing and not enough of another, I've found a recipe that works for me, my husband, my friends and my family. As long as I don't stray too far from that equation, all my boxes stay ticked and I manage to keep on a more even keel – I stay happy being Michelle, I am competent and in the zone as a mother, my work stays in check and Hugh, the centre of my universe, stays in my orbit too.

MY RECIPE

I work out Monday to Friday every day and I make sure I start the day off with 45–50 minutes in the morning – I usually work out with one of the Beeches Mums, Victoria. It's my time and I can think about what needs to be done that day and how I'm going to achieve everything I need to. If working out isn't accessible to you, maybe it's a long walk or taking the dog out; whatever it is, I find I crave some solitude every day to get me set for what might come.

I also need routine and order Monday to Friday. That means all dinners are planned with ingredients in or shopped for, the house is clean and hoovered daily, and the washing basket is empty at the end of every day.

I stay clean with no alcohol and have early nights where work allows it Monday, Tuesday and Wednesday.

Hugh's an early night guy and, other than the weekend, he's always in bed by 10 p.m. We have an early night together those nights and while he's often asleep as soon as his head hits the pillow, we sometimes use those minutes before sleep to chat about issues with the kids or scheduling problems between his work and mine. Once he's asleep, I'll make a couple of lists on my phone: things I need to get from the shops, any kids' party presents if Faith and AJ have been invited anywhere, that kind of thing.

Thursday, Friday and Saturday nights I'll open a bottle of wine. When I'm home, I love cooking, so I'll have a glass while I make dinner and by Saturday night, it could be a bottle. Add to that work nights out, or seeing friends, and it's easy for those units to add up. I'm usually out at least one, if not two, of those nights, either with friends or for work, so they can get a bit boozier than they're meant to. We all do it – we just don't talk about it. Should I cut down? Probably. Will I? Possibly.

I also need some level of spontaneity in my week and usually I manage to get that through work or the Beeches Mums. I love a last-minute invite to something amazing that gives me butterflies of excitement getting ready, or it could be getting the kids from school and driving to see an old friend who's free, or it could be a last-minute invite to an event in London. Whatever it is, I always make sure I leave some space in my week for a spontaneous invite.

Usually on the odd Friday after school, all or some of the Beeches Mums will take the kids to the pub for dinner after school. We might have just one glass of wine, but it means I get through the door at the same time as Hugh, rather than waiting for him to get in and clock-watching until we can start our weekend as a family. By Friday, if I'm in rather than out, I'll make sure I have a couple of bottles of wine in the fridge or Hugh will bring me back a bottle or two on his way home.

Saturday night, if I don't have to go out for work, it means a night in for all of us watching reality TV in our pyjamas and eating sushi with tonnes of tempura. The kids fall asleep on the sofa and we carry them up to bed, and whether it's an early night or a movie, Saturdays are where Hugh and I reconnect.

Sunday has to be a huge roast with the kids, while we spend the day as a family.

As long as I have a mix of spontaneous times, planned time and downtime, friends, work and family, I'll keep afloat. It took me a lot of time, excess and neglect to get to the point where I realised what I needed in order to make my menopausal mind tick over OK.

There are some weeks I can't get the balance right and then I either end up with itchy feet, dying to go out, or dread at the thought of another night out, but I take the rough with the smooth and know that as long as my recipe is kind of bubbling away as it should be, I'll be OK. I take care of all sides of me with a week like this, and that means I'm a better wife, mother, friend and performer.

Don't be scared to experiment with what works for you, just make sure you constantly review your recipe and speak to your loved ones about when they see you at your happiest and when you're at your most relaxed and chilled out. It took Hugh speaking out to help me come to the right balance for me, so ask the people you love in your life what they notice about your behaviour when you're figuring out your own recipe – it'll help you work out what works and what doesn't much faster. Often they'll be better placed to know when you're at your happiest and most serene than you will because they're the ones that will be bearing the brunt of it when you're not.

If it helps, keep a diary of your weeks and rate them out of ten at the end of each one. Slowly, you should start to see a pattern emerge when your weeks are better than others and what those 'better' weeks entail. Whatever works for you, make sure you're working towards something that's attainable too. My perfect week would probably be on a lounger in the Caribbean sunshine but that's not workable or feasible for me, so with reality in mind and obligations and responsibilities in check, develop your own formula.

Don't be too strict on it though, there'll always be things that come up which mean you can't have the same prescripted week all the time; it's about a general sense of well-being rather than a timetable.

CHAPTER 7

Menopausal Mummy: Anger, Confusion and Losing Control

People always say you look for the qualities you don't have in yourself when seeking out a partner, and Hugh and I couldn't be more opposite if we tried. While I've always been the highly strung one in our relationship, Hugh's the even-keel man. If we have an event to go to or if we're meeting friends, I'll leave an hour and a half for an hour-long journey, just in case there's traffic; Hugh will leave half an hour for an hour-long journey, just because he's Hugh... I've always loved a tipple or two; Hugh's never had an alcoholic drink in his life. We've always been polar opposites, but it worked for four years. Until the hysterectomy.

If there had been an identifiable 'first time' that my hormonal imbalance hit us both right between the eyes – if we'd been able to recognise an exact moment, pinpoint it as a direct side effect of menopause – maybe we'd both have stopped, sat down, taken stock and talked about it, or sought some help or counselling. But we didn't. We neither recognised it, nor did we seek help.

What happened in the months following the hysterectomy was the slow attrition of a relationship we'd spent years building. A shift in the dynamic that had worked so well, for so long. While I can't remember in detail the first postmenopausal argument we had, I can remember making the children cry because I was shouting so loud. I can remember feeling so full of frustration, I couldn't stop yelling. At. All.

When the anger comes now, it doesn't come over things that really matter, like Hugh forgetting my birthday, or forgetting to get the kids from school. It comes from him forgetting to put the milk back in the fridge, or something just as trivial. It's almost like I'm Jekyll and Hyde. I can't put my finger on it and I can't prevent it. It's not like any kind of rage or anger I had before menopause. It's new and unexplainable, and I hate it.

It's like watching a storm approach, and knowing you're directly in its path, and you can't stop it coming, you can't outrun it, because too soon you're caught in the eye of it. You just have to let it happen and do its worst. When it bears down on the Heaton Hanley household, there's nothing I can do about it and I know I'll end up apologising for it. For someone who's always been in control, being completely and utterly out of control is a horrendous feeling to try and reconcile.

Any feeling of release, of having got that emotion out, is always quickly followed by a long-lasting sense of guilt and shame, especially if the kids have heard the argument or been in the room. As I sit here in the cold light of day, writing these words, I can't help but feel the kids must notice my change of mood, sharing looks between themselves over dinner, wondering if Mummy is going to get stressed again. I feel ashamed to think that my children might be able to spot when I'm not coping. What lesson is that teaching them? What emotional harm might I be doing to them?

I've pondered it a lot, trying to figure out why the anger feels worse or why the rage takes longer to subside now. I honestly don't know, but I think a bit of it is the fact that as a result of menopause, I feel tired and old before my time, and that's hard to parent through. We're supposed to go through menopause in our fifties or sixties, but I'm in my thirties and I have a young family; it's not a natural combination to experience young motherhood and menopause.

I have some back problems now and I can get injured a lot easier too; both are side effects of being in menopause. I have to make sure I warm up and warm down properly, to reduce the risk of injury, which isn't something that ever used to happen. Hugh, Faith, AJ – they're all young and vital and healthy, and they're a constant reminder that I'm not. And while I know it's not their fault, maybe some of my anger at my situation gets directed towards them.

I have control issues now that I never used to have, too, which manifest in all areas of my life. There's so much of the last six years I haven't been able to control – the physical changes, the emotional upheaval, the recovery periods, the operations themselves – that now, if I find something I can control, I cling to it like a life raft. I control my physique: weighing myself often, monitoring my diet with military precision to make sure it's healthy and using the MyFitnessPal app to make sure I'm on track. I like to control my time in a gym session to the second, and if I have to finish early, it doesn't sit well with me for the rest of the day. I control my external image and always make sure my nails are done, my extensions fresh, my make-up on.

But it's not just control and anger issues either; I get bouts of depression now, which I never had before the operation.

When I'm low and struggling with the darker times, my body manifests my emotions and I feel like I can't move. It's like trying to wade through treacle every day and everything is harder. That can be incredibly tough to parent through, when all I want to do is curl up in a ball and have everyone and everything leave me the hell alone.

I get emails every week from women who tell me they feel the same too. They all talk to me about a lack of energy, an unpredictable anger and control issues that come with menopause that no one really warns you about. You'll be told endlessly about the physical side effects – the hot flushes, the headaches, the dry skin. You'll be told a bit about the changes in hormones, and what that can mean – the sleepless nights, hot sweats. But no one prepares you for the utter exhaustion of some days, when you can't even lift your head off the pillow, but you still have to get to work, parent the kids, put a smile on your face and get through it. In my case, being in menopause with a young family has resulted in behaviours I'll always be incredibly ashamed of.

One spring day, six months after the operation and just weeks before my second injection of HRT was due, as I was loading the washing machine I found some scribbles in pen on one of Faith's T-shirts. It wasn't a top that cost a fortune, it wasn't even her favourite. It shouldn't have mattered, she's got tonnes of T-shirts, but I called her down from her room and demanded an explanation.

'It wasn't me, Mummy, I didn't do it.'

'Faith Michelle Hanley, don't lie to me.'

I could feel the anger starting to build. I was shattered, and Hugh had already texted to say he was working late, which meant no respite for me. I'd felt exhausted all day, but I would still have to bathe the kids and get them into bed, and then make our dinner before Hugh came home.

I was annoyed that Faith was lying to me, and it suddenly became really important to me to get to the bottom of it and get her to admit what she'd done. I should have left it, I should have recognised the fact I was tired and that my emotions were starting to bubble, but I didn't.

'I didn't do it, Mummy, I don't know how it got there, I promise.'

'Faith, go to your room until you can tell me the truth.'

'But, Mummy, I didn't, it wasn't me. I'm not lying, Mummy, I promise. Why are you being so mean?'

Tears started to spill down her cheeks, but her biting back at me was the last thing we both needed. Trying to keep my rising fury in check, I angrily explained to Faith that it was her T-shirt, that she must know how the pen got there and that she needed to take better care of her belongings.

She was sobbing now, pleading again and again that she didn't do it. That it wasn't her. That she didn't know how it got there. Breaking point came, and I snapped, shouting at her to go up to her room. I texted Hugh, telling him what had happened. He texted back immediately, explaining that one of her friends from school had done it and that he'd forgotten to tell me.

Crushed, I crept upstairs, only to hear Faith sobbing into her pillow. I peeped around the open door and watched her blonde curls as her chest heaved and I felt that familiar shame at the knowledge that I'd blown things out of proportion, that I'd been wrong. I'd been wrong to shout and I'd been wrong not to believe her. I knew I was tired and low, and I'd taken it out on my little girl, who didn't deserve it and was too young to understand what I was going through. Hell, I'd been wrong on so many levels, I didn't know where to start. It was just a T-shirt, what did it matter? No one died, no one was injured… Little Faith had borne the brunt of my emotional fallout, at all of four years old.

I gently knocked on her door, tears stinging my eyes.

'Faith, it's Mummy, can I come in please?'

I could see her little head nod, curls tumbling while she stayed rooted to her pillow. I sat gently beside her, stroking her hair, trying to keep my voice even, despite the wave of sorrow engulfing me.

'I'm sorry, Faith. I'm sorry I didn't believe you. I spoke to Daddy and he told me what happened. I'm sorry I shouted at you. I'm sorry, beautiful. I'm so sorry…'

Trying not to sob, I looked up at the ceiling to stop the tears falling. Faith piled hard into my chest, flinging her arms around me.

'It's OK, Mummy, it doesn't matter, I love you. I don't mind.'

I couldn't contain the tears any more. As Faith stopped crying, I started.

While Faith forgave me, it took a long time for me to forgive myself. What sort of a mother brings her daughter to tears over something she didn't do? Let alone the fact I'd lost it over some biro on a T-shirt. I've always had a bit of a short fuse, but until the hysterectomy, until the menopause, I'd been rational with it. Now it seemed my rages were increasingly irrational.

With the children tucked up safely in bed, I told Hugh everything. 'What am I going to do, Hugh? How much of this is me being a cow and how much of it is the menopause? I don't know whether I was like this before because the kids were younger then and different. I'm so ashamed of myself.'

I took a deep breath and bit my lip to try and stop the tears. I'd cried enough after putting the children to bed and while waiting for Hugh to come home; I was completely exhausted by the events of the afternoon and I didn't want to cry any more.

Taking a deep breath, Hugh was honest about his concerns in a way he hadn't been before. 'You know you're not fair to the kids on nights like tonight, Michelle. I can give back. They can't. Today isn't the first time, either. We need to find a solution for all of us.'

He was completely right. It wasn't the first time I'd gone mental over something inconsequential and had to apologise to Faith. The kids won't have done anything wrong or it will've been something minor – they might have spilled something, dropped something, forgotten something; they might still have been in their school uniform hours after I'd repeatedly told them to get changed. But there's irrationality to my behaviour now, and I don't know how to stop it or fix it. Whereas I used to be able to keep a lid on it, I don't seem to have a properly functioning coping mechanism any more – or does this happen to every mum? Sometimes it's normal not to cope so well, isn't it?

I knew it had taken a lot for Hugh to be open and honest with me. He admitted to me that he can tell when I'm having a bad day and when I'm struggling to cope, because I'll send him upwards of nine texts in an hour about how I'm feeling. He knows on those days I need more emotional support than I might normally need from him.

'There are so many days I close the door to go to work and

I know the three of you are going to have a bad day because of the mood you've woken up in, Shell. Some days, you'll be on me and on the kids from first thing in the morning, from before you've even got out of bed, and I'll close the door to go to work and I'll know today is going to be painful.'

'I don't want to be that parent, Hugh. It's a horrible feeling…'

I trailed off, starting to cry again, and Hugh left it at that. I think he recognised nothing he could say would make me feel any worse than I already did and no words were needed to drive home how serious the situation was.

My ability to parent the way I want to has been affected in more ways than one by menopause. As well as the emotional upheaval, there's an increased risk of osteoporosis for women in menopause; I've noticed my back gets put out easier and, once it's out, I take longer to recover because my body is ageing before it should.

My workout pal from the Beeches Mums, Victoria, was round last month and, in a bid to get her daughter out the door after her play date with Faith, she started picking her up and swinging her.

'Please can I have a go?'

Faith was desperate to be swung around too, but rather than asking me, she directed her question at her friend's mum. I knew instantly she wasn't asking me because she knows Mummy can't do those things any more. I've put my back out a couple of times trying to lift Faith or put AJ on my shoulders. The kids know now that if they want to be on shoulders or have a piggyback or be tumbled over and tipped upside down, Mummy can't always do it. It's either Daddy or whoever is closest to hand – in this case, Victoria.

Smiling as first Faith, then AJ queued up to be swung around by my friend, I felt bands of guilt tighten around my chest with my children's every squeal of excitement and giddiness. By the time Victoria and her daughter had been ushered out the door, a black cloud had descended on me and, try as I might, it wouldn't shift. After the kids were bathed and put to bed, I made an excuse to Hugh about getting an early night and lay there in the dark, thinking about what the kids' recollections of me will be when they're older.

I shout, I'm angry, I'm unreasonable; sometimes I can't lift them or roughhouse them. Yes, it's me who keeps the house clean and their beds made, puts food in their bellies, buys their Christmas presents and arranges their birthday parties, but it's Hugh who plays football with them in the park. It's him who puts them on his shoulders so they can see better when we go to Disneyland Paris. Knowing I can't always do these things and that I'm not that mummy always puts me into a very dark state when I think about it, or when it manifests in something Hugh does that I can't. Even writing about it now, I can feel a darkness descend.

There are so many emotions I used to be able to cope with that I can't now. Things that I'd have shaken off a few years ago that stick with me since entering surgical menopause. I get very depressed now, and very quickly, for seemingly no reason or for a reason that just shouldn't be a big deal. I never used to be like that. My emotions are never on a level now, and that in itself is exhausting. It could be something as small as not getting a job that I've gone in for, or not having any work in the diary for a couple of weeks, or a friend being able to swing Faith around when I can't – and all of a sudden, I will feel like the worst person in the world, no use to anyone, for anything.

When I feel that bleakness, that inability to cope descending, there's nothing I can do, I just have to weather it.

While I've never spoken to my children about what is happening, I know it's on their radar that Mummy's emotional state isn't as stable as Daddy's, and that Daddy is way more fun. Faith can see when I get into a moment and she knows not to talk to me, and that's sad. She's only six. She'll say, 'Come on, AJ, let's go and play in your room', because she knows they might start getting shouted at for something that doesn't warrant shouting. Faith can also see that I'm tough on myself too, which is horrible. After the shouting, she's sometimes seen me cry. What am I teaching her about coping with emotions?

I keep everything in, though, and these words will be a surprising admission for Hugh to read, too. I know I have plenty of people I can talk to about that bleakness and how it descends, but why talk when there's nothing anyone can do to fix it? Besides, I don't want to burden anyone with it.

The children both know I've had an operation on my tummy and they know Mummy gets a bad back, and shouty and grumpy, but who cares? They're experiencing me and processing my behaviour through six-year-old and four-year-old eyes and emotions. As they get older, as they reach their tweens and then their teens, they're not going to make allowances in their memories of Mummy. Who thinks about the reasons for their parents' behaviour? No one, or not at least until they are adults and perhaps parents too.

Although I can look at my childhood now and see that my parents must have been affected by money worries and their own sadness at the state of their marriage, my overriding memory of them is of how they were when I was a child, how

I felt as their child – witness to their constant arguments and unhappiness. I'm massively worried that what Faith and AJ experience now could affect our relationship for the rest of my life. Faith and AJ don't care that the way I am at the moment isn't entirely my fault. They're too little to understand menopause and faulty genes, and by the time I can explain it to them, their feelings about their childhoods will be ingrained anyway, and not up for negotiation or redrawing in their teens.

My menopause has affected the kids in so many ways, if I start thinking about them all, it becomes too much to bear.

My Menopause Musings

Menopause is a bit like childbirth, in that no two experiences are the same. Some women go through menopause with only physical symptoms: the flushes, the night sweats, the insomnia; some with emotional symptoms: depression, stress, anxiety; and some go through it with a mix of both.

While there's no 'one size fits all', that's not something to despair about. I spent too long wondering, worrying and stressing over whether I was 'normal' – whether I am 'normal' – in menopause. It's only recently I've embraced the fact there is no normal in menopause, and everyone's experiences are likely to be different.

Don't get me wrong, I hate myself to my very core when I go off at the kids, or when the rage starts to build, and don't think for a second I'm excusing that as 'normal' behaviour. I know it's not. But I can either storm against the way I am or I can try and understand it and learn from it. And while my quickness to anger shows no signs of abating at the moment,

I learn from my behaviours now in a way I didn't when they first started occurring. I'm trying, and while I'm still getting it wrong a lot, it's all I can do.

I've put mechanisms in place that work for me. If Hugh's around and I feel the rage building, I'll go for a workout. If he's not and the school run is over and done with, I might have a glass of wine or call a friend. If I'm struggling, rather than try and carry on, I'll let the kids play on their iPads for half an hour – something which is usually restricted to the weekend. It's not ideal, but it helps me cope better than trying to carry on regardless. only to end up bellowing at them.

My reaction to and emotions during menopause aren't normal, but neither are they abnormal. They're just happening to me, and I can either ignore them, ploughing on and making the same mistakes, or I can try and figure them out as best I can. Of course I wish I didn't feel this way – I'd give anything to feel emotionally like I did before surgery, but I can't. For whatever reason, my resilience is not as unfailing as it used to be, but rather than moping about that fact or resenting it (both of which I do on occasion), I've had to acknowledge it and try and live alongside the new, different me.

I pay more attention to my emotions than I did before menopause, too. I never used to mind or pay heed to when I went off on one, but now I analyse the run-up to whatever meltdown I've had and try and figure out why it happened; try and identify the catalyst that started the chain of events.

For women dealing with the physical symptoms, it might be that they need to look at what they've been eating and drinking before their headache and migraine came, or it might be that they need to be aware of their sleep patterns and how it affects their hot flushes.

Whatever aspect of menopause you're dealing with that feels unbearable, whatever fallout you experience – whether it's shouting at your loved ones, depression, physical symptoms – only by letting it take its course and noticing how you're feeling can you learn from it and put mechanisms in place that will help with it. Don't suffer in silence and don't push on through, telling yourself it'll go away, or that you're stronger than that. Give everything room and space, and learn from it all.

We'll never be the same as we were before menopause, whatever our own individual menopause looks like, so it's about trying to find a new kind of normal, rather than keeping on pushing for an old you that might never come back.

CHAPTER 8

BRCA Babies, Guilt and Dropping the Bombshell

While I can hope the children will understand once they're older what it is we've all been through over the last six years, I'll also have to have the conversation with them about the fact that there's a 50 per cent chance they're carrying the same gene mutation that I do, the one that's meant I can't play with them how I'd like to, that means I can fly off the handle and can be completely unreasonable. They'll have to try and understand one day that they could have the same gene that's made Mummy the way she is.

I'll never be as fun as the other Beeches Mums in their minds because there have been times when I can't swing them as high or as fast as other mummies do. But I'll also have to burden their shoulders with the heavy truth that everything I've been through might lie ahead of them too. It'll be their decision when they get to eighteen to choose whether they want to be screened like I was, or whether they want to live their lives without knowing.

Whether we're right or wrong in how we deal with it, only time will tell, but how do I explain to Faith that her experiences of Mummy being angry sometimes could be what she can expect of her thirties too? That her children's protestations of innocence might fall on deaf ears like hers have on mine too many times? That she might not be able to roughhouse her children if she has them? That if she has children, they might see arguments between their mummy and daddy, like she has seen between me and Hugh?

It's like a double dose of hurt; one they'll look back on and one they might have no choice but to walk headlong into. It's such a difficult and bitter pill to swallow.

Men with the BRCA2 gene mutation have a 1–10 per cent lifetime risk of developing male breast cancer – ten times higher than the general male population. They also have a 15–25 per cent lifetime risk of prostate cancer, which is higher than average, a 3–5 per cent risk of melanoma, a 2–5 per cent risk of pancreatic cancer, and there's an increased risk of testicular cancer too. Although this increased risk of cancer is something I wish AJ didn't potentially face, my main worry for him is that if he carries the faulty gene and has a daughter, he might pass it on to her as my dad did to me.

If Faith has the BRCA2 gene mutation, she, like me, has an up to 85 per cent risk of developing breast cancer in her life, and up to 40 per cent risk of developing ovarian cancer. Those odds won't change in her lifetime; a gene is a gene, and it behaves in a predictable way. If she has inherited the faulty gene from me, science will be the only unpredictable factor affecting the decisions she will have to make.

I have a Google alert set for the BRCA gene on my phone – not for me, but for my children. Faith is all of six now but I follow every development, every news story, in the hopes that if she has the faulty gene, it won't be the bombshell for her that it was for me. There are different news stories every day: increased detection rates from screening; inhibited disease progression from BRCA-related cancers; drugs being licensed in the UK that can reduce the rate of return of ovarian cancer. I read them all, every single story.

Before you think it, I know I might be worrying over nothing; firstly, both Faith and AJ have a 50 per cent chance of testing negative for the BRCA2 mutation; secondly, they've got a couple of decades before it becomes an issue for either of them. All kinds of breakthroughs might have been made in that time that could mean having a defective BRCA gene is as easy to solve as having wonky teeth. Faith might be able to pop a pill, or have an injection, which will safeguard her from all the risks. She might look at my experience with sympathy rather than empathy, as hers might be so different, so much easier, less invasive and less traumatic than mine has been.

My paternal grandmother's journey was worlds apart from mine. She spent the majority of her adult life battling her cancers without knowing they were caused by her genes. Two generations on, I have been able to take preventative action to reduce my risk of developing the disease that Maria fought so bravely against. With that as a frame of reference, who knows what the BRCA landscape will look like when Faith is old enough to choose whether or not to be tested?

We've thought long and hard about how we'll tell her and AJ about BRCA. While everyone will have an opinion on the best way to do it, we've decided a slow drip rather than a bombshell will be the best way forward for our family, our children. Faith's already got an inkling about something – she asked me a few months ago about my boobs, completely out of the blue.

'Mummy, have you had an operation on your boobs?'

Thankfully we were driving home from school, so while

I could see her in the rear-view mirror, she couldn't see my cheeks flush or the deep breath I took.

'Yes, sweetie, you were two at the time, you were too young to remember. Why do you ask, darling?'

'No reason, Mummy, what's for dinner?'

For her, that was it – answer given, conversation over, and she was satisfied. She's still little, and a 'yes' answer doesn't necessarily lead to a follow-up question; she thinks in binary terms and she'd had her answer, but I wanted to see where it was going.

'Why did you ask about Mummy's boobs, baby? You can tell me, it's fine, we can talk about it some more.'

I could see her starting to squirm in her seat – a sign she didn't want me to continue the line of questioning. I wanted to ask again, find out who told her, what they'd said, how she'd felt, but this was about her, and not about me, so I let it lie.

'How does fish fingers, potatoes and sweetcorn sound?'

'Yummy!'

I mentioned our exchange to Hugh that night, after Faith'd gone to bed and we both agreed that all we can do is be open and honest, and answer every question she asks as truthfully as we can.

Sometimes I wish we could know for sure, one way or the other, right now, whether our children have inherited the faulty gene, so we could reassure or prepare them, but the law protects Faith and AJ's choice to make the decision for themselves, and that's right and fair, no matter what Hugh or I may feel. Besides, even if things were different and we could get Faith and AJ tested now, what would be the point?

Imagine Hugh looking at his daughter, knowing she's got

what I've got? That his little, blonde, carefree Faith might have to have the surgeries he's watched his wife go through and struggle to recover from? It'd kill him, and there would be nothing we could do about it at this stage anyway. She couldn't have her ovaries removed before they've developed, no mastectomy.

I don't know when we'll tell her, but it'll have to be sooner than we want to because it's out there on the internet; from our recent conversation, it's clear she's already got an idea or someone she knows has mentioned something. She can already google me, she already knows how to ask Siri for me on her iPad, she only needs to be able to read – and she's getting better at that every single day.

I figure as long as she knows I'm open and that she can ask me anything, those questions will start to come and the conversations will begin naturally. I don't want to pre-empt it too soon, but there'll be people at school who'll talk, and I want Hugh and me to be in charge of the message: what she's told, how she's told and how it's explained for her little ears. I don't want a school friend who's heard something about me from their own mum and dad passing it on to Faith. Kids in her class know who Katie Price is and know Faith's been to her house. Faith's little, and she doesn't know Katie's famous, she just knows her as Katie, her godmother; but other kids in her class talk to her about it. Maybe they're kids with older siblings, who've brought it up, I don't know. It's no big deal who says what when it comes to who Mummy is friends with, but a cancer gene that could shape Faith's future? That's something I want to be in control of her finding out, not the kids at school. It's a terrifying piece of information in the wrong hands, so I want to make sure she's confident in the knowledge of it way before she's at risk of anyone telling her, or scaring her, or relaying the wrong information.

Hugh and I have played out so many scenarios in which we tell the children, the different ways we might phrase things, and – based on their personality types – what their responses might be. They already know Mummy had an operation on her tummy because she wasn't very well. Next, we'll tell them that the operation meant Mummy got better rather than got more poorly. When they're old enough to understand that, we'll explain that Mummy has something in her blood which could make her get ill, so Mummy had the operations to make sure she stays well.

Then we'll have a conversation about their genes, the fact that Faith's big blue eyes that melt me every time I look at them come from Daddy and the fact that bits of her shouty, cheeky little personality probably come from Mummy. That AJ's natural talent for golf comes from Daddy and that Faith's blonde locks come from Daddy too.

Then we'll explain that some of the things that come down to them from Mummy and Daddy are good, but some of them could make you have a tummy ache that hurts. That Granddad accidentally passed down the potential to have a bad tummy ache, so Mummy had an operation so it didn't happen to her.

There's no right age for us to explain this, and we'll be feeling our way in the dark, but whenever Hugh and I talk about it, I feel like I'm drowning in guilt. Even writing about this, I feel filled with remorse and regret that it could be my fault that my little girl has to go through anything comparable to what I've been through.

Having the faulty BRCA2 gene has shaped my entire life since I took the genetic test; if either Faith or AJ decides to have the test as soon as they're eighteen, it could shape way more of their lives than it did mine. I've thought loads about what I might have done or not done if I'd known at eighteen that I was a carrier, and the reality is I know the landscape of my life could have been completely different to the one I live now.

If Dad had had genetic testing sooner, and if I'd found out as a teenager that I carried the mutation, I might not have had kids. I might have decided to have the surgery at eighteen, and my decision might have completely altered the path of my life – no Hugh, no children, a different career, who knows? Would I have had a mastectomy as a teenager? Could I have lived another fifteen years or more with the knowledge that I was at a higher risk of ovarian and breast cancer? I can't say for sure, but knowing my personality type – especially when I was younger – I suspect I might have had these preventative surgeries sooner than I did. I hate leaving things to chance and that's an aspect of my personality I've had since I was a child. If I can control something, know the outcome and not be blindsided or shocked by it, I'll do whatever I can to make sure that's the case. I've always been a bit of a control freak, so I suspect I'd have taken charge and reduced the risk as soon as possible.

I have experience of my journey and mine alone, though. I have no idea what it's like to be told you have the BRCA mutation at eighteen. Will I be able to help my children through the process, if they decide to be tested and to be tested at such a young age? I can only pray that, if Faith is a carrier too, there'll be some other alternative for her than what I've been through. I have no idea how to shepherd AJ through the experience, as a man, if his test results are positive.

I think a lot about the fact that one of the kids might have inherited the BRCA mutation, and the other not. One of them could have it, neither of them could have it or both of them could have it. Of course, if I could choose, I'd want neither of them to have it; but it seems impossibly cruel to think that one of them might be affected, and the other one free of it. One a clean bill of health and a life away from that shadow, and the other faced with decisions, possibly surgeries, that might completely change their life.

There's also their future romantic relationships to consider. Hugh says he would have married me anyway, even if I'd known before we walked down the aisle that I was a carrier. But what if my children's future partners aren't as kind and generous of spirit and love as their daddy is? What if Faith has the gene and a partner says he won't be with her because of the risk to their future children? What if they're not eligible for the NHS screening and what if they can't afford the five-figure costs associated with going privately? What if AJ's partner won't have his children because she won't take the risk of passing on his genes to a daughter if he decides to follow David's path and not get tested?

I spend a lot of time trying to guess whether they have the gene, but the truth is there's no maths or algorithm I can extrapolate from my family history to help predict anything for my two babies. It's not how genes work. If either of them has it, I'll be there a 100 per cent; but it'll be especially tough if Faith has it, because of the surgeries.

I'll always feel like it's all my fault if she has inherited the gene defect, because it *is* all my fault if she has inherited it. Hugh tells me all the time it's not, but of course it is, and nothing he or anyone else says will ever persuade me otherwise. It's the same as the way that I don't blame my dad for passing it to me, but I do still *have* it because of him, and he blames himself for that. That's a complicated way to feel, but if my two babies turn out to be carriers, whether they blame me or not, I'll always blame myself. However I feel about it, though, the conversation needs to be all about the children; I will have to put my feelings of guilt aside, because it'll be about helping them choose the right path through the diagnosis, looking at every available option and being the rock to them I so desperately needed when I was diagnosed.

While I approach it all very emotionally and get upset at the prospect of possibly having dealt the children the hand I was given, Hugh's far more matter-of-fact about it and refuses to let me wallow in guilt or feel blame. Whenever I mention it to him, I get the same pep talk he's been giving me since Faith was a baby and I found out about BRCA. It goes something like this:

'I'm not being funny, Shell, but you need to man up. It's not like you'll have chosen to pass this on. If either of them has it, we just have to deal with it. It won't be your time to cry. It's out of your control, so there's no point in feeling guilt about it. The BRCA2 gene issue isn't a lifestyle choice, it's not like you've done anything wrong that's meant you have this faulty gene, there's physically nothing you can do. It's impossible to feel guilty for an outcome you can't have controlled. Absolutely impossible. You might as well blame yourself for the sun rising or setting every day.'

But no matter how many variations of the lecture, pep talk or whatever you want to call it I hear, if my children have inherited the BRCA gene mutation, I'll always feel guilt that it is because of me.

While the children are my responsibility, my brother David isn't so much. Mum's desperate for him to get tested – I was on the phone to her a few months ago when she brought it up for the umpteenth time with me.

'Michelle, will you speak to our David? I've talked to him about getting the test done and I know he said no at first, but I honestly think he's coming round to the idea. Can you have a chat with him? He'll listen to you and he'll think I'm nagging if I keep going on about it.'

After a few texts between us later to check if he was free to chat, I called my little brother and he knew what the call was about straight away.

'Has Mum been on at you to talk to me about that bloody gene again? I've told her I'll make an appointment, but I'm not sure about it now. I didn't want to when we found out because it honestly didn't seem like a big deal. I know it is for you but not me, right?'

'You're kind of right, my risks are higher but I could have passed it onto Faith and AJ.'

'Yeah, but Shell, I'm single…'

'I know that, you dope, I'm being serious. You can get genetic screening now which means if you found someone mad enough to have kids with you, they could be born free of the gene. That's how far science has come in a few years.'

'Seriously?'

'Yes, seriously. David, I know you don't want to and I don't know why, but don't make any daughter you may parent have to go through what I've been through. Knowing I could have passed that gene onto Faith and AJ is something I think about every day and that's completely avoidable for you.'

'You have had a shitty journey…'

I couldn't tell whether my argument was persuading him.

He's always been headstrong and likes to be in control of all his own decisions – just like me.

'The thing is, Shell, even if I find out now, there's no preventative surgery for men to lower the risks. I'd find out and be powerless to change anything. Right now that's not something I want to do. Call it ignorance, call it whatever you like, but for me I'm not sure it's the right thing to do. You know I'm single at the moment, if I'm in a position when I'm in a long-term relationship to start a family I'll re-evaluate it then. Of course I don't want a daughter potentially born with this thing if it's avoidable, but all of that's a maybe and a long way off…'

'So what shall I say to Mum? Because she's going to call me in a bit and see whether I was able to persuade you.'

'You can tell her it's not a no forever, it's just a no right now. I know how hard things have been for you and I don't want to see anyone else I love go through what you have, especially if a genetic test is available to prevent it or screen any potential children I might have for it. If by some miracle I settle down and want to start a family, I promise I'll do everything I can to make sure my kids don't go through what you've been through. That OK?'

'Deal.'

While I hope my brother does get the test, with all my heart I hope at least one of us is in the clear…

My Menopause Musings

Passing on a potentially deadly gene defect to your children isn't a position any parent wants to be in. Genetics are completely in control of whether Faith and AJ have the faulty BRCA2 gene, and it's going to be a long, drawn-out waiting game to see if the guilt I feel constantly when I look at them is merited or not.

While I want to be there and support them, it's ultimately their journey too and they'll be in charge of how much or how little they share with me. If Faith tests positive, I can't demand that she tells me her plans; whether she'll have a mastectomy, whether she'll use genetic selection if she wants to have a family. None of that is my business. If she has inherited the faulty gene from me, then ultimately it becomes her gene and how she handles living with it will be her decision.

I did what I did and what I felt was best for me, but I can't say it's best for everyone and if – like some women with BRCA I know – she decides against surgery and opts for watchful waiting and monitoring, I will have to respect that decision, even though it's not the one I chose for myself.

I've read so many articles and visited so many forums and taken so much advice on board about how to have the conversation with my children, and what to say. All I can do is support her and AJ as much as I can and be here if she ever wants to talk.

CHAPTER 9

Married to the Menopause – Aren't I Entitled to Be a Bitch Sometimes?

In July 2010, when BRCA was just a set of letters to me, I walked towards my future on a sandy beach in the Bahamas. Having been together since 2008, when we met in a Dublin nightclub, Hugh Hanley and I said 'I do' with only the priest and the photographer as witnesses. It was a beautiful ceremony, and one that we enjoyed sharing together as a newly married couple. We then came back to Dublin and celebrated in style with 100 of our treasured family and friends.

We promised to love, cherish and honour one another in sickness and in health... We took our vows seriously but had no idea then that 'sickness' would mean 'preventative invasive medical procedures to reduce cancer risk', which wouldn't have tripped off the tongue as easily during the vows.

There are millions of couples in the world who walk down the aisle thinking they know what the next fifty, sixty or seventy years of their life will bring, only to have it turned a little upside down. We're in by no means a minority at having our 'happily ever after' revised after the fact and on a sliding scale. I know what we've been through is nothing compared to what some people have to live with.

If Dad hadn't been genetically tested, Hugh could have been looking at raising the kids alone. But despite the knowledge that my surgeries have greatly improved my chances of being around for Hugh, and for our children, for many years to come, with each operation I have felt less womanly; less like the woman my husband took as his wife on that sunny day in the Caribbean.

I know not every woman who has been through what I have will feel the same, and I know plenty of women who'll wholeheartedly disagree with me – that's fine, and I completely respect their thoughts and opinions. But for me, my internal female organs and my own breasts were a huge part of what made me feel like a woman, which is something I didn't realise until they were taken away. When I said 'I do' to Hugh, I had my own boobs, the ability to bear children, no scars, and the fruit of life at my fingertips – now that's all gone. In a nutshell, I feel less like the Michelle Heaton my husband married.

These nagging feelings have resulted in significant confidence issues; where I used to scrape my hair back and not bother, I now feel the need to emphasise my femininity to compensate for the organs I've had taken out of me. I've had some amazing conversations with women who feel completely differently to me, though, so I know I'm maybe in a minority.

I've changed myself irreversibly, both emotionally and physically in order to hopefully be around longer for the people I love, but that's inevitably come at a cost. While we'll never have any more biological children, there's also the cost to the physical attraction that so much of my relationship with Hugh has been based on. Has our sex life changed since I underwent a mastectomy and hysterectomy? Yes, if I'm being honest, how could it not?

No one had told me about what would happen after the mastectomy and reconstruction in 2014, but the truth is I have no feeling in my boobs whatsoever. No sensation where there used to be plenty. I know every woman is different and sensation loss varies from from one woman to another, but my truth is that I have no sensation at all.

While my boobs might be more pleasing on the eye and to the touch to my husband, when we're being naked and intimate, there's no sensation there for me. I had limited feeling post-operatively and that's decreased now.

It must have taken me six months after the mastectomy to let him touch them too. They didn't feel like mine, and being intimate with Hugh felt like he was touching a foreign body. It wasn't nice, but you don't consider these things when you're reducing your risk of breast cancer and potentially saving your own life. You don't think about the little implications – and in the grand scheme of things, this is one – but they matter. Every single time he touches me there I'm reminded of BRCA, reminded of my surgeries and reminded of the bombshell that went off in our family.

Every. Single. Time. I'm sorry, Hugh.

I didn't tell him the truth about not wanting him to touch my boobs after my mastectomy because I didn't want him to feel differently towards me and I hoped some sensation might come back, but it didn't.

For a couple who had always prioritised a physical closeness as much as an emotional closeness, it wasn't easy for either of us. I think Hugh noticed a reticence on my part, but we were dealing with so much, he always gave me the physical and emotional space I needed while reminding me he was there if I ever needed to talk about anything.

I could have, maybe should have, sat down and been honest with him. I know these words will come as a shock for him to read. But I didn't want to tell him because I didn't want him to feel awkward when he touched me, so for over six months after the mastectomy and reconstruction I came up with excuses as to why he couldn't touch my boobs. I'd tell him they were sore or that I'd banged one and felt a bit bruised, I'd tell him my scars were itching and annoying me, I'd make up every and any excuse I could so he wouldn't touch the pretend boobs I now lived with. The ones in my body that weren't mine.

He never pursued it, never demanded anything, and never got upset at my continual rebuffing of any advances towards my chest. He'd hold me close, tell me he loved me and soothe me until we fell asleep in one another's arms. I suspect he knew there was an underlying issue, but he never pushed it, instead preferring to wait until I was comfortable enough to talk about it.

Thankfully, our emotional connection hasn't changed since the day we got married, but physically our lives will never be the same again. My boobs still feel incredibly awkward and when he does touch me there, I pretend that it's fine when it's not. It's one of the oddest sensations and really difficult to describe. I can see him touching my boobs but I can't feel it despite the fact it's my skin and my body. I can feel if his hands are warm or cold but that's it, no sensation, no tingling or goose bumps like there used to be, and I hate the fact that element of our physical relationship is gone forever.

But it's not just my boobs that feel different – my entire

body and what I see when we're intimate is different, and that's changed everything. When we have sex now, all I can see is scars. The once womanly frame that wrapped around him on our wedding night looks and feels aged and changed. And because that's what I see, my confidence in my body when we're intimate has plunged lower than I ever thought possible.

I have a slight apron of skin where I split my staples in the weeks after the hysterectomy too, and while Hugh doesn't care and loves every inch of me, I see it every time I'm naked and it reminds me of everything we've been through.

Lots of women who contact me have a full-on flap of skin, an overhang they can't shift that puts them off having sex with their partner, and while I try and get them to see something positive in their reflection, the truth is, more often than not, I struggle to in mine. If all you see are the imperfections, it doesn't matter what anyone else says. Hugh tells me all the time I turn him on and I see that when we're intimate, but I don't feel as sexy and I don't look half as good as I used to when I'm naked.

There's a guilt I feel about obsessing about it, though; after all, I'm here, I don't have cancer, I'm alive. But there are so many physical aspects of the menopause we don't talk about; my sex drive has been one of the major issues for me post hysterectomy, and yet there's very little help available to women feeling like I did and sometimes still do now.

Google 'hysterectomy side effects' and you get 2.4 million results, the majority of which talk about emotional, mental and hormonal changes. There are physical changes mentioned, but they're things like headaches and urinary incontinence. A lack of libido comes pretty far down the list, if at all, yet if the women who stop me in the street or at the supermarket are anything to go by, the physical side effects are the ones they have the hardest time dealing with, the ones that go on to affect their relationships.

I should have spoken to my doctor about my flagging libido way sooner than I did. I battled it for a year before I had the courage to raise it as an issue. I'd think about bringing it up at every appointment but wouldn't, hoping it'd change on its own and come back to a level like it had been before the hysterectomy. When I finally had the courage to talk about it, there was a simple resolution, a change to the oestrogen-only HRT I'd been on since the operation. I'm now on testosterone and oestrogen, which has put it back on track but if I'd 'fessed up sooner that it was a problem, I could have had the solution a lot sooner too.

But it's not just the want for sex that's changed in menopause; I don't behave in a way I used to during sex either. I was never a 'hanging from the chandelier' type of woman – for me sex has always been about a deeper connection and a strong emotional as well as physical bond – but there used to be an abandon in me with Hugh, which isn't there now. I'm constantly trying to hide the parts of myself I don't like, which means things aren't as natural as they used to be between us when we're intimate.

Of course every married couple expects their bedroom habits to change over time, but there wasn't a gradual evolving change with us, it felt more like a juggernaut grinding to a halt. Sometimes I make excuses about why I can't be in certain positions because I don't want him to see my scars, for them to be a focus for him – which I'm sure they wouldn't be – but it's more about me. I know he's seen it all before, he was there when our babies were pulled out of the same hysterectomy scar but it didn't bother me as much then as it does now. After children, that scar made me feel capable and confident; after the hysterectomy, it made me feel empty. I'm gradually changing how I feel, but it's a process and it doesn't happen overnight. I'm trying to see them now more as battle scars where I dodged a bullet, but it's a slow shift in perspective.

Hugh's been nothing but supportive throughout the whole process but, while I know every woman's husband or partner is different, one of the many things that's been hard for him is my ever-growing need to unburden myself and his frustration at not having solutions. Whether it's emotional baggage, physical trauma, anxiety at work or how I look, I've gone to Hugh with issues that he's found hard to hear because he thinks he should have an answer, when all I really need is an ear. I've explained several times that I don't need him to have a fix for everything and that I just need to share some of what I'm feeling, but he's a pragmatist and, in his eyes, if there isn't a solution there's no point going round and round and talking about it until there is.

But it's not just the physical and emotional aspects of our relationship that have changed. While I shout at the kids sometimes, Hugh has become an emotional punchbag for me and that's not fair on him and definitely not what he signed up for. I'm a moody cow and I flip off the handle a lot, often over nothing. We've never gone to bed on an argument and we've never walked out the house, but we've always had different approaches to confrontation and those differences have been exacerbated in menopause. Whereas I always like to clear up disagreements there and then, Hugh will walk away and take the heat out of the situation, then come back and hope cooler heads prevail.

For me, whether it's World War Three or an apology and

back to normal, whatever the resolution, I need it to happen straight away, and sometimes a resolution can be hard to find when it's World War Three and the situation has gone nuclear. There've been one or two arguments over trivial things that have led me to throwing the remote control at a wall, in a bid to release the white-hot rage that has descended on me. I don't know how else to describe the anger in moments like that – it's a complete shift of mental state and I feel like I've lost control of a situation. Luckily I have a husband who doesn't rage back, because if he didn't deal with it by walking away and cooling down, I don't know where we'd be.

We had an argument last week that started with him buying the wrong vegetables for dinner on his way home. It shouldn't have been a big deal, but it was, and it completely changed what I'd planned for dinner.

Does it matter in the cold hard light of day?

No.

Did it matter at the time?

Yes, it was the worst thing he could have done and I couldn't let it go. I started with a few comments about how it ruined dinner, and then it escalated to me calling him useless, that he couldn't even remember and get the right vegetables. I shouted and ranted while he busied himself putting them away and clearing away the kids' dinner plates, and when I paused for breath, he spoke quietly: 'You're being ridiculous, Shell; what you're doing and how you're speaking to me is completely unacceptable.'

He always says something along those lines, and if I'm still in a rage then I'll shout back at him, but if I've got it out my system, I'll be devastated and I'll cry. That day I sobbed from the bottom of my heart.

'I'm so sorry, Hugh, I don't know what's happened to me. I'm a bitch, you should leave me, I'm sorry for the way I treat you. I don't know where it comes from, I don't understand myself.'

Sometimes he'll forgive me and sometimes he'll say, 'Sorry is just not good enough any more, it's ridiculous.'

Just last week, almost out of nowhere, a few days after the vegetable episode he said, 'Shell, sometimes you talk to me like shit, you've got to change.'

We talked about my emotional volatility a bit and while he didn't say anything in a confrontational way, I knew he wanted to help me and get to the bottom of why I behave the way I do, because it has an impact on the kids and on him.

'You're right, I do talk to you terribly and you know I'm always so sorry after I've flown off the handle. I know I'm doing it; I can hear it but I can't stop, it's like verbal diarrhoea.'

What brought him to the point of telling me he'd had enough? Working out. He said he'd train with me the following day, and then said he felt guilty he wasn't seeing his friend for a gym session. While my kind and caring husband was just trying to keep his wife and a really good friend happy at the same time, my tolerance was zero and rather than say, 'It's OK, we'll train another day, darling', the rage started to descend.

'Just let me know whatever you decide.'

He could tell from my terse tone that it wasn't going to end well.

'Yeah, but if I did that, Shell, you'd be annoyed.'

'Hugh, sometimes you need to be a man and make a man's decision and stop asking my permission. Just man up a bit.'

'Michelle, where is this coming from? I am a man.'

'Well, just man up then and tell me what you're going to do.'

'Shell, if I told you anything you'd have a go at me for doing what I wanted. You're so unreasonable sometimes, I hate you when you're like this.'

His comment was utterly justified. He was right, he couldn't have won in that situation, and it hit me hard, like a verbal slap across the face. An instant guilt overwhelmed me. Hugh – as always – had just been trying to do right by everyone. He didn't want to let me down because he'd promised he was going to work out with me and he didn't want to let his friend down, who he owed a gym session to, and I'd ripped into him because he was trying to be kind to both of us.

He walked away from the dinner table without waiting for me to finish – a sure sign I'm in the bad books – and seconds later I could hear him upstairs, getting ready for bed. I'd pushed it too far and he didn't want to know me, much less make up. I cleared away the plates and loaded the dishwasher, and by the time I went upstairs and got into bed, he was lying with his back facing me.

'I'm sorry, Hugh, I really am. I don't know why you're with me, you could do better, I know you could. Can you forgive me? I'm scared you're going to leave me… I'm scared one day you're going to say it's all too much, that I've changed too much and that you'll be happier without me. That the woman you married is gone.'

He rolled over in bed, sitting up on his elbow.

'Shell, I'm not going to leave you, I love you. You're just a bitch sometimes, and I hate it.'

With that he rolled back over and left me in the darkness with thoughts that kept me awake most of the night.

I've never blamed my moods on hormones or the menopause, though, because I don't know that's the reason. Is it the hormones or am I just being an absolute cow on that day? I don't know and there's no way to know. By the same token, and to look at the other side of the coin, why can't I be moody or grumpy sometimes without everyone thinking it's the menopause? I'm entitled to be pissed off if I've burned dinner and anyone who's ever been in a mood knows sometimes you snap out of it and sometimes you don't.

I get that some of my moods are unreasonable, but they can't all be, can they? Surely I should be as entitled as everyone else to get the hump and be in a mood about things that happen sometimes? But I try my best not to be because, firstly, I don't know whether it's really me, the real Michelle, being in a mood or whether it's something to do with hormone levels; and, secondly, how I deal with being in a hump is different now. It's involuntary, and those reactions aren't always the best.

It's an easy excuse to blame my hormones but is it the right one or the lazy one? Yes, maybe my hormones are to blame for a lot, but maybe everyone would feel the same way I do if they were in whatever situation I'm in. Who can say? I have a friend who constantly asks me, 'Are you feeling hormonal, love?' whenever I'm in a mood, and it always annoys me because it feels so patronising. But the truth is I'll never know whether she's right or I am. The very second I had the operation to remove my ovaries, Mr Sheridan inserted an oestrogen implant, so technically I've never been without hormones. But whatever it is, my emotional stability isn't what it used to be and no one can tell me why. That's what must be so hard for Hugh to cope with.

Did I used to be like that? I've always been hot-headed but I was never as bad as this. I've changed emotionally since the operation – perhaps it's the cumulative toll of receiving a life-changing diagnosis, having two babies and undergoing two major body-altering surgeries in the space of two years. But try as I might I can't find a way back to how I used to be. Like I'm in the woods and the trail of breadcrumbs that I left behind me has disappeared. Tall trees surround me, and there's no way back.

I'll catch my reflection mid-rant when I'm on one with Hugh, and I'll think, 'Oh my God, what's wrong with me? Why am I like this? There's nothing wrong with my life.' But I can't stop the anger.

I'm always either full-on up or down, always on a pendulum swing, and Hugh never knows who's going to be at the door when he comes home from work. It must be equally exhausting for him as it is for me. But do I make allowances for that? No, I don't, even though I should. I've got the best husband in the world; he's always put his family first, there's nothing he wouldn't do for us and I return that love and compassion by yelling at him and pushing away the physical closeness he's worked so hard to keep in place in the face of everything.

There's a depression that I never had until I went into menopause too. Don't get me wrong, everyone gets down, I know that, but I didn't suffer the dark moods before like I have since the hysterectomy. I feel like my emotions are more prevalent since the menopause. I'm definitely more weepy, and I cry a lot more than I've ever done at any other point in my life. I feel so low sometimes that no matter what happens and whatever joy I have in my life at that time, I can't shake that feeling of darkness. It's like someone is holding my chest. Crushing it. I feel so low and so depressed. Faith could have got a gold star at school or AJ could have been dry through the night, I might have just got a great job or an audition I've been dying for. Whatever joy arises in my day, it doesn't matter – if I'm low, I'm low, and nothing will pull me out of it. Some days I wake up and I feel like the unluckiest person in the world.

It's like a switch being turned on and off randomly; I can go to bed so down and then I'll wake up like nothing has happened, or the opposite can happen, where I'll go to bed happy and contented, then wake up like the worst thing in the world has happened, despite the fact I've been asleep for seven hours. An entire book could be dedicated to mood swings and emotions during menopause, and while I've tried my best to explain mine, I know from the women I speak to that everyone's are different. It seems the one thing we all have in common is that they're exhausting, both emotionally and physically.

I'd give anything to go back to the old me for a few months, the one who still enjoyed highs and lows and flew off the handle but the one who was measured, who was able to keep emotions in context and not be owned by them so totally.

I can hope as my menopause journey continues that the mood swings will be easier to deal with and that I'll start to gain some control over them. I will be on HRT until I reach fifty or fifty-one (the usual age that women naturally enter menopause), which means I could be looking at another twelve years of this and that's an exhausting thought just to contemplate for myself, let alone trying to figure out how my marriage will withstand it or what state it'll be in afterwards.

While everyone's emotional experience in menopause will be different and their arguments with loved ones individual, there's science that backs up the symptoms of mood swings in menopause, especially the lows I and the women I speak

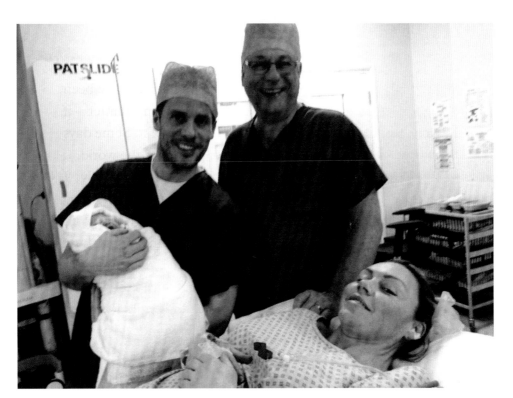

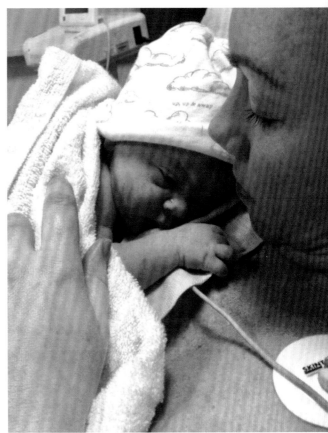

Above: With Hugh, my gynaecologist Mr Sheridan and my gorgeous new boy, AJ, just after his birth, 24 February 2014.

Right: Being unable to breastfeed my new baby was a shattering experience.

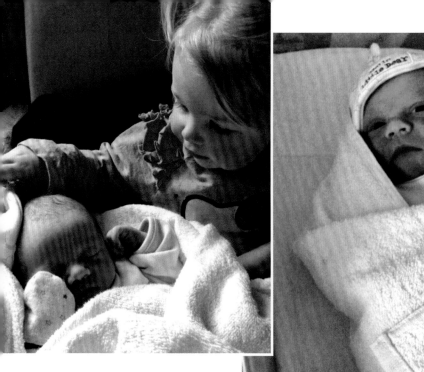

Above: Faith meeting AJ for the very first time.

Below: Soon after he was born, little AJ was back in hospital with meningitis. When he came out of hospital, his big sister, Dr Faith, didn't want him to get sick again.

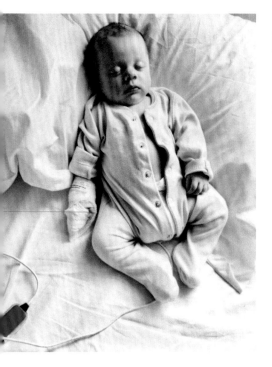

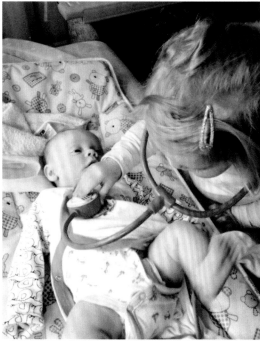

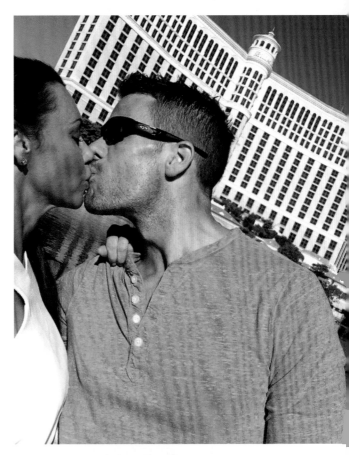

Right: With Hugh on holiday in Las Vegas before the hysterectomy, 2014.

Below: The morning after my hysterectomy.

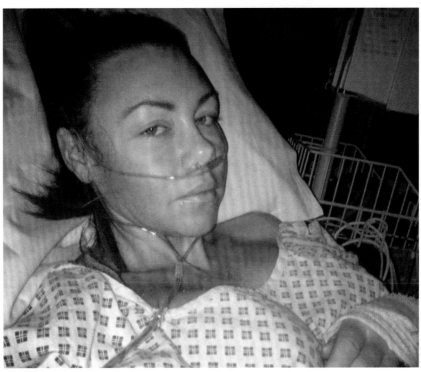

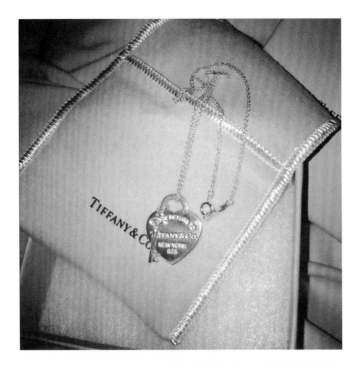

Left: The Tiffany necklace Faith brought into the hospital for me.

Right: My scar, a few days after the stitches came out, uneven due to me working too soon after the operation.

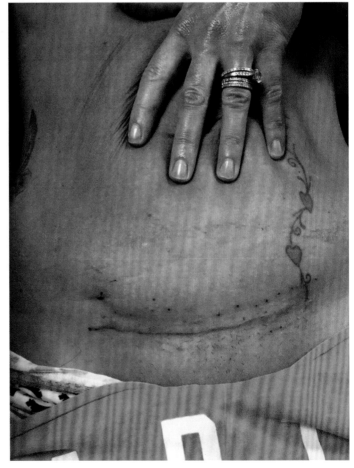

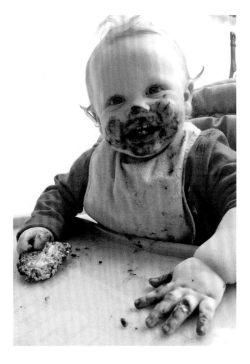

Left: AJ at one year old. It's impossible not to smile at this picture.

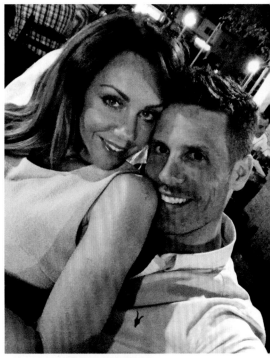

Right: With Hugh in Cyprus for my friend Rochelle's wedding in June 2015.

Below: The Beeches Mums on our first night out together in 2016.

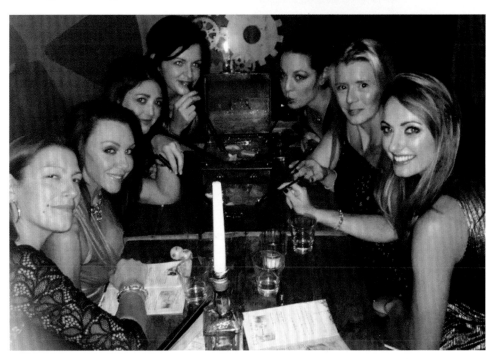

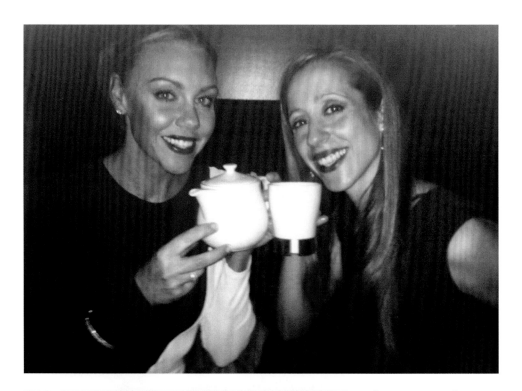

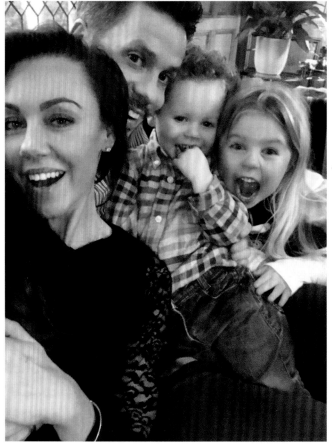

Above: Cup of tea, anyone? With my friend Vivianna on a night out in summer 2016.

Left: The Heatons' family Christmas in Ayr, where I was in panto in 2016.

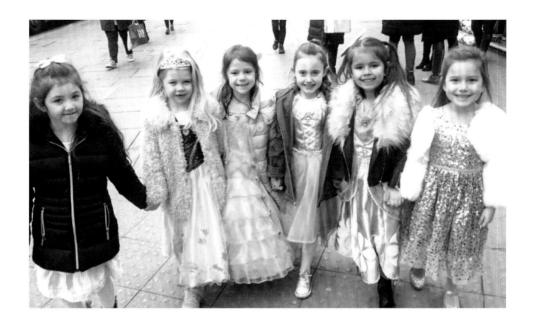

Above: Faith with her best friends (all daughters of the Beeches Mums) on Faith's sixth birthday in 2018.

Below: AJ, with pure delight on his face, at his fourth birthday party, 2018.

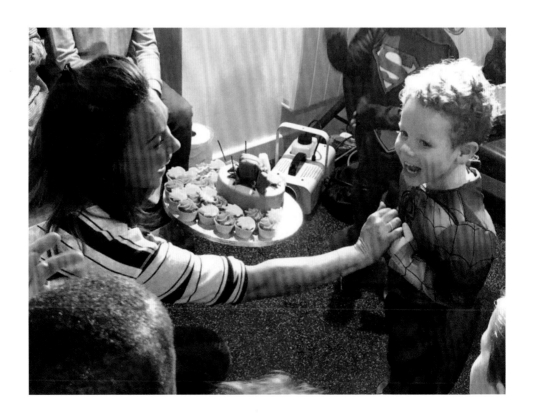

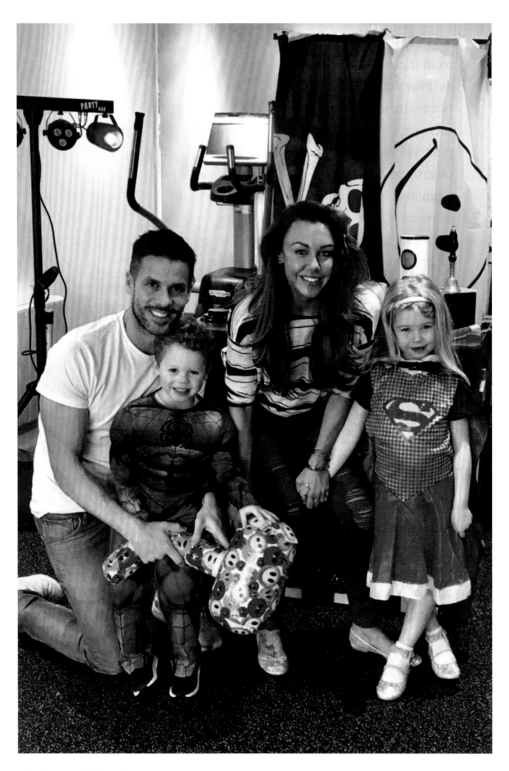

My beautiful family.

to in the street seem to suffer from. Mood disorders are twice as prevalent in women as they are in men and they often occur during periods when hormone changes are happening: teenagers entering puberty, women during pregnancy, post partum and in menopause. The relationship between oestrogen and mood is a complex one which varies from woman to woman, but the depletion of that mood-regulating hormone during menopause should never be underestimated and there's a lot of work being done by scientists with bigger brains than mine to try and figure it out.

I didn't and don't ever excuse my behaviour by blaming the menopause, but if I had made Hugh more aware of a link between the two from the beginning, things might not have escalated as often as they have. Hugh knows there's a connection between menopause and mood, but I don't think he understands how inextricably linked my menopause and mood are. While I'm going through this, so is Hugh and so is our marriage. All we can do is keep trying to do better and understand it more.

I speak to him about what's happened after I've flown off the handle or after I've been really low but it doesn't excuse it; all the sorrys in the world don't make it better or make my behaviour OK. I've improved a lot since the early days and I've got to continue working hard to keep things more in check. My marriage could ultimately depend on it and I've lost enough in the last few years – the thought of losing my husband too is something I can't even contemplate.

Hugh's Menopause Musings

Is Michelle the woman I married? Of course she is, but I'd be lying if I said our marriage hasn't changed since she had the hysterectomy. Both physically and emotionally, Michelle's a different woman now. Until recently, though, I never factored the menopause into her mood swings as much as I should have done from the beginning.

Whether I didn't think to in the heat of the moment or whether I didn't put it down to that, I don't know, and while I do think sometimes I should be more patient with her than I am, sometimes (and she's the first to admit it) she's just a bit of a bitch. Sometimes the children haven't done anything wrong or I've just got out of bed and, those times, we don't deserve the approaching storm, no matter what Michelle is going through. When I can clearly see she's woken up like that, I try and stay out of her way and give her some space. I'll avoid the grief however I can because, ultimately, I just want the easy life, a good marriage and happy kids.

Having talked to her at length about what you're reading right now, though, I only know with hindsight that I went into Michelle's hysterectomy as ill prepared as she did. I saw it as a regular medical procedure, a straightforward operation: she'd have it done, there'd be a recovery time and then she'd be OK, and life would carry on as normal, we'd all pick up where we left off. Of course I was told Michelle would go through menopause – but everyone presumed I knew what menopause was. How am I supposed to know that, as a guy?

No one offers the husbands or partners or kids counselling at the time of a hysterectomy and because I didn't realise the scale of the emotional impact and fallout of the procedure, I didn't do any of my own research until fairly recently, which meant I wasn't maybe as tolerant in the early days as I should have been.

We weren't taught about menopause at school, it wasn't part of sex education in Ireland, and having spoken to guys about it when Michelle's been stopped in the street, I'm not in the minority either. It seems there are plenty of blokes out there who go into their partner's menopause with as little preparation as I had.

I knew there was a potential change of emotions and maybe hormones, but I honestly didn't know what that meant and I didn't know how that would manifest in Michelle or our marriage or her parenting. I've realised since talking about this that I need to learn more about the menopause and that's three years down the line. I could have been better or made things easier for all of us by familiarising myself with what it meant – both immediately and in the future – in the run-up to the surgery.

But I didn't.

I put shutters down, and I need to bring them up.

Menopause isn't something you get over for a long time. It's going to be with us all for years, there'll be more emotional changes to come, I know that now, and because of the circumstances and the age Michelle was when she went into menopause, hers is going to last a lot longer than it does for most women.

Michelle is never one who flatlines, it's one of the many reasons I love her – she's highly strung, and with that comes an amazing passion for life, and when her energies are channelled right and she's in a good place, she's infectious and one of the most incredible people in the world to be around. But when it doesn't align, she can be impossible to live with.

She's always been up and down and she's always been the fiery one – I knew what I was getting when I walked onto the beach all those years ago – but since menopause, those feelings and emotions have been magnified and she's not as in control of them as she used to be. I can see she's trying and she's constantly evolving and learning from all the outbursts, but it's a marathon, not a sprint, and I can't expect everything to go back to normal quickly.

If someone at work told me their wife had the faulty BRCA2 gene and was going to have the same operations as Michelle has had, in the past I would never have spoken about the challenges of the immediate emotional state straight after the operation, but I definitely would now.

Nine out of ten times when she shouts or rages, she gets over it. Once or twice it's lingered, though, and as she's attested here, I'm not afraid to call her out on it, no matter how angry or upset it makes her. I wish it was as easy as her telling me what to do and how to make it better, but she can't because she doesn't know. I hate that she's trapped in this cycle of emotional volatility and I'm completely unable to help her get out of it or deal with it.

It's exhausting for her but both of us having spent a long time talking about it, our concerns are more for the kids and what they see when she gets into one of her rages or depressions. It's impossible to know how much of it could potentially be down to hormones, though, and how much of it is dealing with having a young family and the stresses that come with that. Comparatively speaking, very few women are going through menopause and raising a young family at the same time, and the truth is that the kids have made menopause a million times harder. Any parent will tell you their kids push their buttons, but combine Michelle's vulnerable emotional state into that and things get harder.

I know that if I googled 'menopause' then the mood swings would come up as a symptom, but we also didn't have kids before; take the M word out of it for a second, children are their own kind of hard. If we take Michelle as a 100 per cent, then I don't know what percentage of her behaviour is down to her being in menopause, what percentage of it is down to the fact she's parenting two little people while I'm at work all day and then working in the evening herself, and how much is just what she's like as we're both growing older and changing.

Even discounting the menopause and the hysterectomy and the BRCA2 gene issue for a minute, the Michelle we know and love now and the one from four or five years ago are different, but we've all gotten a little bit older in that time, we've all changed in our own ways. I see a change in me since the children arrived, it's the sheer pressure of having them; parenting is a constant job, so it's hard to dismiss the way Michelle is purely as the menopause.

I've seen her get down a lot more since the menopause, which hasn't been nice to see. Before she was the iron woman and incredibly strong and emotionally resilient. Her Twitter name is @WonderwomanShel and I always call her Wonder Woman. Nothing used to get her down, nothing would beat her and if she did hit the deck for a while, she'd be straight back up and in the ring as quickly as she could be. But seeing her get low now is really hard, especially because I'm her husband and there's nothing I can do to get her out of it or help her find her way back. I can't find her in that forest and, try as I might, even if I could, I don't have the trail of breadcrumbs to help her find the way back out either.

She masks a lot of what she's feeling with anger, though, and that's hard to navigate. She can shout and blow up at me and then afterwards she'll admit she's been down or depressed. Life would be easier for us all if she were more honest with her emotions and if she let them be what they are, let them have their day, rather than trying to hide them or suppress them. She's always been incredibly hard on herself and she's even harder on herself now. The tougher it is for her to understand her emotions, the tougher she is on herself, which isn't easy for me to watch.

I'm trying to adjust how I react to her anger. At the start I'd have bitten when she was in a rage, whereas now I know it'll pass and I take deep breaths, and check in to see she's OK. I'm trying, but I still don't understand the emotional aspect of the hysterectomy, I didn't when she had the surgery and I don't really now.

It's hard seeing her get so upset. Things get to her that wouldn't have bothered her in the past. But I just have to be patient and wait for the strong Michelle to emerge again. I don't think we've nailed communicating about it, though. She doesn't talk to me when she's having a bad day; I just end up in the firing line. But I hate negativity and when I come across it in life, I just remove myself from it. If there's ever a negative issue in my life, I walk past it, but I can't do that with menopause so we constantly have to adjust to it in our lives.

I didn't do any of my own research when Michelle was going in for either of her surgeries, because at the time I thought it was the right thing to do – I figured I'd rather not know what the side effects were. The way I saw it, I'd just deal with them as and when and if they happened after each operation. I don't like worrying about what might come in the future as Michelle has already mentioned; as a result of being the way I am about things, I probably wasn't as supportive as I should have been, which put a bit of a gulf between us at one of the most important times in our marriage. Even when we got the information about BRCA, I didn't research it. I stepped back and let Michelle make the decision herself. We chatted through the options and I fully supported her, and we talked about it a lot, but I let Michelle be the one who researched it and then I backed her 100 per cent in her choices. My attitude was always, 'She's got to live with it, it's got to be her that's happy with the outcome.' I'll always be a sounding board, but I've never wanted to push an agenda or suggest what I'd do if I was her. All I've done is offer the support I swore I would do when we made our vows.

When you marry, it's for better or worse, and this has got to be chalked up as part of the journey we're on together. Yes, we've gone through a hard time as a couple, as parents and as a family since the mastectomy and the menopause, but we've dealt with it as best we can and we've learned from every aspect of it, as hard as it's been to come through. We're not a 'what if' kind of couple, we deal with what's put in front of us and I for one tend not to worry about things I can't control.

I know one thing though, for a fact: I couldn't have gone through it as well as Michelle has and one of the first things I'd suggest any partner or husband do is try to walk a mile in their wife's shoes, because it's not easy. I wouldn't have been brave enough, I'd have chickened out of the operations definitely. She's far stronger than I am. She's the rock in our family and while that rock sometimes has slightly craggy bits, she holds us all together emotionally.

The fact she willingly went into hospital perfectly healthy to have parts of her body taken away when there was nothing wrong with them was an exceptionally brave decision to make, and one the children will be immensely proud of her for when they learn about it too.

As her husband, there've been really hard times, not just post-operatively, but in the run-up to and on the day of the surgeries themselves. Her hysterectomy was incredibly difficult. I was in a heap when she went through the doors to surgery, and the minute those doors closed I cried buckets for my beautiful wife.

There was nothing I could do to help, not a single thing I could do to make a difference. It caught me hard and it knocked me sideways. The doors closed and I couldn't help her at all.

Every marriage or relationship is different and every menopause is different too, but I wish I'd shown more tolerance, I wish I'd understood sooner the seriousness of what Michelle was putting herself through emotionally. I wish I'd researched things myself and I wish I'd made Michelle be more honest with me. I wish I'd pushed her to explain how she was feeling more and I wish I'd made more allowances. I know I'm not great at communicating, but even writing her a letter explaining how I felt or asking her to write one to me could have helped us communicate better.

I tell her all the time I'm proud of her and what she's been through, but I know she brushes it off. I wish I'd made her listen and I wish she really knew and believed how amazing she's been. Every time she's stopped in the street, it makes her emotional because she doesn't think what she's done is incredible. She sets such high targets for herself and her standards are so high, I wish she'd take a minute and look back at how far she's come, rather than how far she still has to go in front of her. She's carried herself with dignity while she's battled to find a way through it all and she's tried to keep us all as unscathed as possible. Even when that hasn't worked as well as she'd intended.

If you're the partner of someone on this journey, do your research, increase your tolerance levels and communicate however you can. It's what will keep you together as you try and navigate your way through menopause as a couple. Educate yourself. Learn everything you possibly can about what menopause is like and what changes and experiences are common. I found this out the hard way and we clashed over some silly things when I didn't spot the signs and understand what she was going through.

Once you see that mood swings are part of it and that it's nothing you're doing, you can relax about her ups and downs. I had to learn to be patient. Patience is vital in both the short- and long-term. Cutting her some slack when she seems sad or angry will go a long way.

And most importantly, while there may be bad days, where you feel like you can do nothing right, remember why you're together. She is still the woman you married and love, so man up, support her and help her through it. She needs you now more than ever.

CHAPTER 10

Hot Work and Lack of Confidence

I remember talking through my decision to go public about BRCA and my mastectomy with Hugh and my mum before I did it. I knew I'd look different after the operation; my surgeon had told me he couldn't recreate the boobs they'd remove. I'd be out of work for a while, I'd be in hospital, recovering… I knew it'd come out somehow, and I wanted to control the message and tell it my way – without drama, just with honesty. It felt like an issue that needed to be out there and while I didn't particularly want to be the one talking about it, the thought that it might help others was important to me. I figured maybe telling my story on the platform I have might help others in some way feel less alone and isolated than I'd done when I found out I had the gene.

Lorraine Kelly's team filmed me on the run-up to the mastectomy – while I had genetic counselling, while I met other women who'd been through the journey I was about to embark upon – throughout the day of the surgery, and also my recovery. The response I got from women who watched the shows was incredible and helped me massively. Every tweet, message, Facebook post and email to my agent made me feel like I'd made the right decision in sharing my experiences. Talking about my hysterectomy and menopause came naturally after having talked about my mastectomy, and I'll always be grateful to the *Lorraine* team for giving me that opportunity.

So many women I speak to don't have the luxury of speaking out and being honest. I met a woman recently who told me she felt her hot flushes had halted her career in its tracks. She didn't have the courage to go for a promotion she'd been asked to interview for because it entailed several meetings with her bosses, and her hot flushes were holding her back because she didn't want to experience one during an interview. They were so intense that sweat would pour down her face, dripping off her nose, and the thought of that happening at a vital moment was too much to contemplate, so she decided to decline the offer of interviewing even though it sounded like she completely deserved it.

I have no idea where she worked, but it broke my heart that her workplace environment didn't feel like a safe space where she could talk about it. There was no boss or member of HR who she felt she could be honest with about what was stopping her from going for the job.

By law, employers have a responsibility to be aware of menopause but very few are. This woman was just one example of the many women who've told me being in menopause has held them back in the workplace. My industry isn't different to any other either, in that I've been held back by it too.

Half of the UK workforce is made up of women and there are currently 3.5 million women workers over the age of fifty in the UK. Consider the fact that the majority of women go through menopause between the ages of forty-five and fifty-five, and roughly speaking that means there are millions of working women going through it right now who are turning up daily to offices, schools, hospitals and workplaces across the country. Are they supported? If the women contacting me are anything to go by, the answer is not enough.

Unison guidelines say menopause is an occupational health issue but research from the British Occupational Health Research Foundation says workplaces across the UK are routinely failing women in menopause. Their report, based on speaking to nine hundred women in menopause in the workplace, found half of the women surveyed hadn't disclosed they were in menopause to their workplace and that where women had had to take time off work to manage the symptoms, only half had revealed the real reason for their absence to their line manager. It's a completely normal process every single woman in the world will go through, so why are we lying to our employers and why don't we feel able to be honest about it?

Half of the women questioned said they'd tried to negotiate flexible working to manage the symptoms but had been refused and, heartbreakingly, three quarters of the women on HRT in the study said work was the main reason they'd started taking it – in the vague hope of managing their symptoms better.

Another study from the Trade Union Congress surveyed five hundred safety representatives in different workplaces across the UK on menopause and found 45 per cent said their managers didn't recognise problems associated with menopause.

While all these figures make for sobering and depressing reading, they are a loud and clear wake-up call that the treatment of women in menopause in the workplace needs to change dramatically. That managers, workers and employers have a responsibility to increase and improve awareness for a condition that every single woman in the UK is going to go through. Menopause is a longstanding health condition and should be treated as such by employers. Mental health is legislated for in the workplace, why not menopause?

There've been recent calls for employers to do more for employees in menopause, with suggestions that it should be treated much the same as pregnancy and legislated for in the workplace in law.

A 2018 BBC survey interviewed 1,009 women between the ages of fifty and sixty, all of whom were in menopause. It found that 70 per cent of the respondents hadn't told their bosses they were experiencing symptoms; a third hadn't visited their GP to get any help; and nearly half of them said the menopause had affected their mental health.

Another 2018 study from King's College London tracked 124 women in menopause in the public and private sectors. The researchers found a programme of cognitive behavioural therapy delivered in a self-help book dramatically reduced the extent to which women found their menopausal symptoms problematic.

There's a seismic shift starting to happen in terms of how we view and talk about menopause, but it's not happening fast enough and there are millions of women in the UK who are still being failed daily by their workplaces. It's not acceptable any more. Menopause is one of the least sexy words in the world, I get that, but it's time to change.

Think about it, when was the last time you saw the word in a headline or mentioned in a TV show or as part of a soap plotline? When have you ever heard someone talk about it on the red carpet? No one wants to hear about it or read about it, yet we're all going to go through a version of it in one way or another.

I made the decision to talk openly about mine, but it's come at a cost to my career, which has changed since I decided to be open and honest about having the BRCA2 gene mutation. Google my name now, and the fact I've had a hysterectomy and am in menopause is the fourth link you'll come to. Never mind all the other things in my professional career I've been able to accomplish.

I've been lucky I haven't had to have the painful conversation with a line manager or boss, though – that's something I'm incredibly grateful for. I was able to control my story and the messages from it; other women I've spoken to aren't as lucky. The women I've met on my journey all tell me that admitting they're in menopause in the workplace is painful and embarrassing and if that wasn't bad enough, it seems there's very little – if any – understanding, compassion or sympathy out there for the condition.

I don't have a regular set of colleagues, I meet new people and I work with different people all the time. While you can find out I'm in menopause if you search the internet, barely any of the people I work with know I'm in it. The minute it comes up or the second I tell them, people look at me in a different light and I hate it. I'm tired of menopause being in the shadows and something we're all supposed to keep quiet about, not talk about.

There are no popular songs or poems about it, there aren't any movies about it, even newspapers and news channels only report on it once in a blue moon, when someone famous mentions it or – like Angelina Jolie – someone has the preventative surgeries I did if they have the BRCA gene, or another medical condition, such as endometriosis.

While initially I thought my industry would be great in helping me to bring awareness about menopause, in all the conversations I had with Lorraine and other TV hosts, all the interviews I did for *OK!* and other magazines and newspapers, I didn't for one second factor in any effect it might have on my long-term career. After all, despite my surgeries and my condition, I can still sing, dance, learn lines. It was a procedure I'd been through, not who I was – why would it have any impact?

I couldn't have been more wrong and within months of the operation, I started realising I wasn't getting booked for the same kinds of jobs I used to get booked for. Something had changed, and it took me a while to realise that me being linked to the menopause was it. I wasn't getting the sexy campaigns any more. I used to get booked for food campaigns – once I sat in a bath of yogurt as part of a sexy shoot for the Yogurt Week campaign; another time, I'd been photographed for No Carbs Week, where I'd ripped open a loaf of bread dressed as Cindy Crawford. But now, these types of brands weren't coming knocking any more, or if they did cast me, they'd change their mind at the last minute and one of my peers – a singer or a footballer's wife – would get the campaign instead. Literally the only difference between us would be the fact that I'm going through the menopause and she's not. Like somehow the fact I couldn't carry children or get pregnant any more had robbed me of my womanhood or my ability to be sexy.

I spent a long time upset about it before that upset inevitably turned to anger at being overlooked when, professionally, nothing had changed about me at all. The relationship between sex appeal and menopause is a difficult one to decipher. Women in their fifties are still sexy – a glance at the red carpet at the Oscars tells us that. So why does talking about menopause instantly reduce that sex appeal? It shouldn't, but it does.

There's a metaphorical scrapheap, and it feels like you're added to it when you go through menopause, that your best days are behind you, but that's not the case for any woman I know who's going through it. I'm fighting hard not to end up on that menopausal scrapheap, but it's a constant battle. Hell, there shouldn't even *be* a menopausal scrapheap, but there is.

Menopause is a physical process, but it doesn't have to change who you are or what you're capable of doing professionally. The reason I've written the book you're holding in your hands is because it's time the rhetoric changed and I want to be at the fore of its evolution. I feel like I have an incredible opportunity as a menopause pioneer – which I'll admit isn't a terribly snappy title, but it's the truth. If I'm going to be put in a menopause box then I'm going to get out of it, stand on it and use it as a soapbox, to shout as loudly as I can. I need to bring people in to my world. Menopause is an experience I'm working through; it's not my entire existence.

I know both from my own experiences and from those of the women I've spoken to, finding understanding from colleagues can be hard to come by too. I did a job recently where I was with the same people for several weeks while we worked in close proximity. While I was on that job, something came up in the news where my menopause was mentioned, and while my colleagues were all supportive and said a sentence or two about it, from that moment on, no one invited me out on the equivalent of the after-work drinks and everyone talked to me slightly differently. It was still with respect and they were still very kind, but it was akin to how you might talk to an old school teacher if you saw them in the street, or your parents' next-door neighbours from when you were a kid.

I don't blame them; menopause is the elephant in the room once people know you're going through it, no one knows what to say. Suddenly other people feel like they have so little in common with you that you're basically unrelatable, so you're left there lingering, exactly the same person as you were five minutes ago, but suddenly viewed completely differently.

I don't want anyone to try and relate to what it's like to be in menopause, you can't possibly if you're not. I want people to try and relate to me, Michelle, for who I am, not what I'm going through.

Why can't I be sexy and in menopause at the same time? There shouldn't be any rules that stop me being both, but society makes me believe that there are. Opinions won't change overnight, but if every woman in menopause had one conversation a week about sex appeal with someone else, a whole army of us would mobilise and start changing opinions across the world.

As Hugh will attest, though, when I want something or when I feel something strongly, not much gets in the way of me airing my thoughts or striving to get what I want, and that's one thing menopause hasn't changed in me. Society doesn't think menopause looks like me, so that's the perfect starting point for me to deliver the message that menopause doesn't look how any of us presume it does. It's individual, and it doesn't change us completely.

Menopause doesn't mean wrung-up, dried out and finished. Far from it. There's a whole swathe of women going through surgical menopause, early menopause, perimenopause (the period shortly before menopause) – does it mean we can't do our jobs or does it mean we're not invested in our careers? Of course not.

I guarantee you the next time you set foot outside your front door or walk through your local town, you'll pass menopausal women. We're everywhere and it's down to all of us who are in menopause to shout louder, bang the drum, talk openly and say: 'This is what I am going through, it's not who I am.'

I've spent long enough angry about the way working lives can change during menopause, though; I've spoken to too many women frustrated at not having the courage to go for the promotion or too scared to tell their boss the real reason for their day off.

Going live in a bikini on *Loose Women* in 2016 was the start of my fight back. I was terrified of doing it, but it was my line in the sand. I was scared stiff and shaking like a leaf, standing there in a bikini, talking about my scars and the operations I've undergone, but the response I got was overwhelming.

I'd been booked to appear on the show and I had a phone call the afternoon before. I knew they wanted to talk to me about my scars and what I'd been through in menopause, but what came from the producer next wasn't at all what I was expecting.

'We know you're probably going to say no, but we're going to ask you anyway because we think it'd be a really powerful message: would you consider doing the interview standing up in a bikini and literally talking the panel through your scars and how they've affected you and what they mean for your body confidence?'

'In a bikini?'

I wanted to check I'd heard correctly and when I realised I had, I politely declined. I'm no different to every other woman out there when it comes to social media – we all put the best version of ourselves out there, but with cameras on me from all angles and harsh studio lighting, there wouldn't be a 'best version'.

It'd be me, scars and all, in broad daylight, for everyone to see.

I wouldn't be able to smooth down my skin or point a camera from an angle where my legs looked longer. Every shot would capture the skin rippling, the loss of elasticity, all of it.

But while I'd originally refused the request, I couldn't stop thinking about it when I hung up from the call. It wasn't that I objected to the request or the premise, far from it. In fact, there was something about it that struck a real chord with me. It was still playing on my mind when Hugh came through the door a few hours later. I told him what they'd asked of me and told him I'd said no, but that I couldn't shake the idea from my mind and while he didn't say I'd made the wrong decision by saying no, after we put the children to bed and were having dinner, I asked if he thought I was doing the right thing by turning it down. His answer turned into a pep talk (as Hugh's conversations often do) and completely changed my mind.

'Michelle, you're telling people to be positive every time you do an interview about your journey. You're telling women it's possible to overcome surgery or whatever life has thrown at them, that whatever they've been through doesn't have to own them, that they can move past it and move forward. You talk all the time about how menopause won't hold you back professionally, how you want people to talk openly about it, how you want to use it as a springboard to make women feel confident about themselves, whatever they've been through, whatever their size, whatever their scars. But how can they move forward if you can't? How are they supposed to feel confident if you're not setting the example honestly? I've seen the tweets and the messages you get and reply to, you're always telling women they can be strong and be proud of their bodies regardless of what life has thrown at them, but how can they be if you're not? How can they follow your example unless you set that example first?'

Less than twelve hours later, I appeared on screen for the first time in a bikini in menopause. I told Ruth Langford on the show how I felt it was important for women to feel more confident about their bodies no matter what size they are. I talked about the fact that no matter what our bodies look like or what they go through, we can all do whatever we want to do and all be whoever we want to be.

My whole body was shaking by the time I was finally given a robe, having stood there showing my scars and talking about menopause to the nation for over three minutes. It was both terrifying and one of the most exhilarating things I've ever done in my life. The thousands of comments and tweets both I and the show got confirmed that my husband had been right. There wasn't one negative comment from anyone about what I'd done.

While some said they admired me, there were plenty that brought tears to my eyes, telling me that seeing how nervous I was made them realise that to move forward you have to push yourself out of your comfort zone, no matter how hard and nerve-wracking that is to do.

It'd be easy for me to stay in the menopause box, to give up and put the bikini away, dress differently and accept what my body is going through and transition into a different part of my career. But I won't. It's not fair to me and it's not fair to the millions of women like me who still have so much to give, despite what their bodies are doing.

I refuse to accept the premise that menopause makes me 'past it' professionally, physically, or in any way. I've got more energy some days than most of my younger friends, I'm usually the last one out with the Beeches Mums and they're all younger than me. I'm not ready to grow up. I've got more to give and I won't stop until I've given it, regardless of what my body is going through.

Menopause can happen at any age; I've heard from teenagers in menopause, and they've got the whole of their working lives ahead of them, trying to adjust to it. Working when you're in menopause can be knackering, exhausting and frustrating – even without having to factor in bosses or an environment which doesn't support you or understand what you're going through. Whatever physical symptoms you're dealing with in menopause, they're all very difficult to deal with at work, especially if you're in a customer-facing role or if you work in a place where you're not allowed to open windows. Every single woman in menopause, no matter her age, deserves to spend her working life in an environment where it's not hushed up or ignored. We all deserve to work in places where we're not embarrassed by what's going on in our bodies, where we're understood and where we're as celebrated as everyone else on the team.

But it's not just the physical symptoms that can rear their heads at work. The emotional fallout during menopause can make work feel unbearable. When I get my down days, nothing can bring me out of it. I'm exhausted, depressed, I cry at the littlest thing and really struggle to hold myself together. If I have a show to do, or if I have to travel to India or Dubai for work or for a job, for example, I can't call and explain I'm emotionally vulnerable and need to rearrange it. I have to go and I have to be who people expect me to be. Putting on that mask can be incredibly difficult and emotional, it's exhausting, but like millions of other women working through menopause, when you have professional responsibilities you stick to them and you meet them, menopause or no menopause.

Being in menopause affects my confidence levels too. I've always been self-deprecating and have never revelled in my talents. I'll always explain away the fact that I made it into Liberty X by saying 'Oh, my face fit', or 'I was just lucky'. I'm not the most confident of people on my best day, so when I'm feeling emotionally vulnerable and I have to rehearse for a show with Atomic Kitten or for a panto, or with the Liberty X girls, I can find it really difficult to be the best I know I can be. My belief and self-worth are low at the moment, and while I'm not striving for perfection, I do want to be the best I can be. When I don't feel strong, I'm harsh on myself and beat myself up. I just want to be good enough and so much of the time I don't feel good enough. I want to be good enough at everything – at parenting, cooking, cleaning, singing, acting, working, dancing – and I very, very rarely feel like I am.

These feelings of increased anxiety that I experience now also change who I am at work. I was late for a shoot a few months after the hysterectomy – it wasn't a huge deal; it was some casual headshots. There wasn't a massive team waiting for me, no studio being paid for while I ran late; whichever way I cut it, it just wasn't a big deal and by 'late' I mean less than five minutes. But the second I knew I was going to be late, I started panicking and crying. I couldn't cope with the anxiety over someone waiting around for me and me costing them some of their time. I was a blubbering mess by the time I got to the shoot and had to wait ages for my eyes to stop looking red and sore before we took the pictures. It shouldn't have been a big deal that I was a few minutes late, but for me it felt like the world was ending. My professional life is ruled by anxiety now, in a way it never was before.

I've never met a woman who's used menopause as an excuse, though, and I would never presume I can wheel out the fact I'm going through it to get out of something I don't want to do – hell, I nearly killed myself sticking to work commitments just days after my hysterectomy. No menopausal woman wants a 'get out of work free' card, we just want some understanding and support from our employers, and a working environment where we're not judged or demoted or overlooked for a promotion because of what we're going through physically.

Workplaces need to recognise and support women in menopause because the reality is that if they don't, they're leaving themselves open to employment claims on grounds of corporate workplace responsibility and discrimination, not to mention the fact they're overlooking a whole army of women who have dealt with more than many people could ever imagine and yet keep on fighting.

My Menopause Musings

Whether you're at the start of your journey or in the middle of it, if you haven't told your workplace, now is the time to do so. It won't be easy, but without them knowing about it they can't support you.

You have rights as an employee going through a long-term health condition and those rights need to be upheld. If your industry has a union and you're happier talking to them in the first instance, that's fine, but you need to start asking for help if you need it or if you feel the symptoms of menopause are holding you back. Arrange a meeting with your line manager and get HR along too, and see where you go from there.

In terms of the day to day, and working while dealing with menopausal symptoms, there are things you can ask your manager and workplace to accommodate which could reduce the effect the symptoms have on your working week. While this list isn't exhaustive, it might help for a start:

Uniforms
Synthetic uniforms can exacerbate sweating, which is something that already increases during menopause. If your uniform is synthetic, there may be another option or you could be moved out of a customer-facing role for a while.

Desk position
Are you next to a radiator or an open window? Having control over where you sit can make a difference in coping with symptoms of increased sweating, hot flushes and chills.

Temperature
Is your office always the same temperature? If so, who decides that temperature? Can you ask them to accommodate your needs by adjusting it to alleviate your symptoms?

Drinking water
If there isn't a water cooler, do you have access to cold water or a fridge in which you can keep your own supply?

Flexible working

Do you have to start and finish at the same time every day? Flexibility can help you cope with sleep problems and night sweats.

Toilet breaks

Are these limited during your shift or working day? If so, speak to your manager about relaxing the rules in your instance.

Colleague awareness

Rather than hiding your menopause from your colleagues, tell them what you're going through. Explain the symptoms they may see in you and how they manifest, whether that's mood swings, or tearfulness, or other behaviours that seem out of character. Understanding will breed tolerance.

I'm fortunate that the majority of my menopausal symptoms are emotional rather than physical. I don't get the hot flushes, the headaches that my mum suffered from for decades, but I'm in the minority and the reality is that most women in menopause will be battling physical symptoms daily in their workplace. While employers have a responsibility to legislate for those issues, we, as employees, need to make sure we're talking more openly about what's going on.

I didn't take the details of the lady who stopped me, the one who decided she wasn't going to go ahead with the offer to apply for a promotion. I wish I had, because her story stayed with me and made me feel incredibly passionate about the working rights of menopausal women.

I like to think she changed her mind and went for the promotion and landed it but I'll never know.

CHAPTER 11

Moving Forward

Only recently has there come a point on my journey, from finding out I had the faulty gene to having a mastectomy and hysterectomy, where I've been able to stop, draw breath and try and be proactive rather than reactive. Since 2012, life has been one reaction after another: raising Faith, having the mastectomy, getting pregnant with AJ, having AJ, his meningitis, the hysterectomy, the recovery. Like a ball in a pinball machine, I bounced and careered wildly from one operation to another, one recovery to the next, never having the time to properly stop, gather myself and my thoughts, and prepare for the next step on the path.

But there came a point around a year ago where I was finally able to exhale and think properly about the future, rather than continue to react to the present. Where I was at last able to think about looking further forward than I have done for a very long time.

While AJ's only four, he's getting older and a little more self-sufficient with each day; he's not a baby any more. Yes, we still have a young family, but they're growing up and their needs are changing.

My life has a routine to it now – or at least as much of a routine as it can have, given the job I do. For so many years, I've felt under attack, both physically and emotionally.

I battled to reduce my risk of breast cancer, fought to reduce my risk of ovarian cancer. Tried my best to recover as fast and as well as I could, and get back in the saddle as quickly as possible.

I'll always have the faulty BRCA2 gene and the reality is there's a small chance I could still get either one of those cancers. But I'm over the worst now and I've done everything I can to be around for a long time.

I'm learning from what's happened to me so far too. My marriage has survived and I believe we're over the worst, but I've got a lot of learning to do and I'm still adjusting. While I had a small amount of genetic counselling at the beginning, I'm trying to come to terms with what the last six years have brought to my family, and the truth is there's an element of trauma that I'm still struggling to get over. No one's built of steel, even if I like to think I am. I'm not unbreakable, and I've come close to breaking point too many times to mention in the last six years. I prided myself for years on having a high level of mental and emotional resilience; it has taken some adjusting, now that some of that resilience has gone.

I can contextualise a lot of things, but finding out I have the BRCA2 gene mutation and the journey my family and I have been on has been the hardest thing I've ever had to deal with in my life. Pretending it hasn't changed me is foolhardy – of course it has – but those changes don't have to be negative ones and, if they are, it's about finding the positive in those moments and times and learning from them.

I've always been able to deal with the big things in life – the operations, the recovery, my finances – but things are harder now. I've still got that resilience, but I have to dig deeper for it now, it's not on tap. Are my reserves just low at the moment, will they build up again? Or has menopause changed me that much that it's taken some of my fight? I don't know.

I know that small upsets can feel like the whole world ending. Having said that, though, I have never once felt like I was completely broken; I've felt close to it and on the ropes hundreds of times, but never down for the count. Thanks to Hugh and the journey we've both been on, we're definitely looking to the future, but I still have to reconcile the past and this book is part of me trying to do just that. To recognise it, give it some space to breathe and be, and move on.

I can see how lucky I am with my life; my family is amazing. I've got a lot to be thankful for, and I don't want to feel sorry for myself, but I feel sorry for the people around me who have borne the brunt of this journey so far and who have steadfastly loved me and kept me going through it all: my husband, my children and my family.

I get incredibly upset when I talk at length about menopause and what it's meant to me, so this book has been a truly emotional journey to commit to print. It's been very healing and I've learned a lot about myself in the last six years and writing these words.

I'm more resilient than I thought I could be, I've also learned I need to communicate better and be more honest about my real emotions with my husband. I'm trying to be kinder to myself, too, because the reality is this something I could be dealing with for at least another decade or even longer.

I can't envisage a time at the moment when I won't be on HRT and while it's been a lifesaver and prevented me from having many of the menopausal symptoms other women I know suffer from, I've still got a lot of adjusting to do, because the Michelle who went under general anaesthetic twice isn't around any more. But rather than mourn for her, I've got to start being kinder to the Michelle who is around.

I'm trying my best to be a better mother, I'm trying to extend more patience, to plan better so I've got play dates lined up which might mean my weeks aren't so hard emotionally. I'm trying to count to ten or remove myself from a situation when I feel the anger descend. I'm trying to recognise it and see where it comes from. I'm trying to be honest about it and I'm trying to figure out whether it's really anger or whether it's upset or fear or worry that I'm masking as something else.

I'm also trying to binge less, I'm packing my schedule with professional commitments and while that's its own level of exhausting, it leaves me unable to get into negative eating and drinking cycles, because I need all my energy for work.

I'm trying to take stock of what's been a lucky escape, too.

Yes, I've endured surgeries, had complications and am in menopause, but I could be living with cancer. I'm incredibly fortunate I found out about BRCA and was able to have the preventative surgeries before cancer had a chance to occur. Many BRCA stories I hear aren't as lucky as mine has been. The cells they took away during my mastectomy came back clear, with no precancer in them, and the cells they took away for analysis during the hysterectomy came back clear too.

I dodged the bullet. I've been lucky.

I've found three or four lumps on my breasts and have had them biopsied, but I've been incredibly fortunate so far and none have turned out to be anything sinister.

Ovarian cancer symptoms are similar to IBS, which I can suffer from, but I'm constantly vigilant for any change and know what to do if I ever find anything I'm worried about.

But while all of that focuses on the positive, I'm still aware in the back of my mind that while I might have eliminated a huge proportion of the risk of getting cancer, I haven't and I can never eradicate it completely. There'll always be a risk I could still get breast cancer and, while I don't have ovaries, there's still a risk of female-specific cancer. Despite not having ovaries I still have some risk of ovarian cancer. The figures are much more manageable now, though, and much easier to stomach. I'm down to around a 2 per cent risk for breast cancer and around a 3 per cent risk for ovarian cancer. There's a chance they could have left some cells behind, but I'm now very low risk, so in that sense, for now at least, the surgeries that have been so tough have been worth it.

I've spent a long time in the last few years wondering whether I'd make the same decisions again, if I'd had a crystal ball to see what happened to me, to my marriage and to my family – whether I'd walk the same path again. I wish I could change many things about the last six years, but I do know I'd make the same decision as I'd made all day long. Definitely. I watched my grandmother go through it because of this faulty gene we both share, so I know nothing I've been through is as tough as what I could be facing.

I've got a lot of making up to do to my Hughie too. He's put up with so much, I'm lucky I haven't lost him. We've been married almost eight years this year and I've pushed him as far in the last few years as I think I ever will in our marriage. While writing this book, Hugh asked to watch the *Loose Women* clip of me in my bikini, talking about my scars. He's been an integral part of helping me write this, not least with his own musings in Chapter 9. He hadn't watched the segment before, not because he was uninterested but because he'd been at work when it had aired. He knew it had been an incredibly emotional thing for me to do, so while he'd said he wanted to watch it whenever I was ready, that moment only came a few weeks ago.

I was as nervous watching it back as I had been doing it, especially knowing Hugh was watching it too. I didn't know he was intending for us to watch it, but after I came down from saying good night to the kids in bed, it was teed up and ready to go on Sky Plus.

'Hugh, what's this, what are you doing?'

'I never watched this and I figure you're almost at the end of writing the book, so now seems as good a time as any to watch it. I know it was the hardest thing you've had to do so far on this journey and I'm proud of you for it, so I thought now was a good time to have a look. You don't mind, do you?'

You could have heard a pin drop in the lounge while we watched it, and I could barely breathe, much less look at him. I've never needed approval from anyone but knowing Hugh thinks I've done the right thing is always important to me. As the credits aired, I had tears in my eyes and turning to him I could see he had them too.

'Shell, I don't know what to say...'

He gathered me up into his arms and held me tightly.

'I knew it was an emotional day for you, but I didn't realise how much strength that must have taken. You bared all and you spoke honestly. You've been like a brick wall these last six years, you've stood there and taken everything life and BRCA have thrown at you. I know you haven't found adjusting to life now easy and I know you're down on yourself about how emotional it's all been and how difficult it's been for all of us, but I honestly couldn't be prouder of you. Talking like that has taken such strength…'

He paused to pass me some tissues, having felt my body wracking with sobs in his.

'It's done now, Shell. We can move on; we can move past it. We've ricocheted from one thing to the next for the last six years and we've been through more in those years than most marriages go through in a lifetime, but we're coming up for air. I love you, I'm proud of you and I'm glad you're my wife…'

For someone who isn't always the best at communicating, my husband's honesty and his words that day meant the world to me and have stayed with me. Whenever I feel things are tough, I remind myself of who I have standing shoulder to shoulder beside me.

In bed that night, as he spooned me while we fell asleep, he told me again how proud he was of me.

'I can't wait to look back on all this when we're old and reminisce about the hard time in our lives and how we came through it…'

'Hugh, I don't want to look back and reminisce about this, I want us to be the couple that constantly looks forward to the good times we have ahead of us. We've had enough hard times behind us, maybe it's time we look forwards and leave the past where it should be…'

We're on the menopause journey together but we're adjusting to what it's brought us so far, and I've learned a lot about myself and my relationship along the way. I'll never be one to congratulate myself and give myself credit for what I've been through in the last six years. It wasn't bravery; for me, it was necessity. I've irreversibly changed myself physically in order to hopefully be around for longer for my husband and children, but I don't dwell on what I've done and it'll never feel like something I deserve credit for. Why should I pat myself on the back when I don't see self-worth? I do stuff like yell at the kids, give Hugh a hard time for no reason; while I continue to do things like that, I won't celebrate anything, because I'm not the finished article yet. I hope to be one day, but I'm not yet.

A few weeks after Hugh watched *Loose Women*, our daughter Faith turned six. Her birthday parties have evolved from when she was four and while the Beeches Mums and their little ones are all integral to the celebrations, we usually arrange a night out after the party for the mums to decompress.

I was clearing away plates and filling up squash jugs when I caught sight of the birthday girl hovering in the background. She was twisting her hair and seemingly waiting for me to finish what I was doing so she could have my undivided attention.

'Faith, are you OK?'

'Mummy, what operation did you have on your tummy?'

With the noise of her sixth birthday party in the background, I wasn't sure I'd heard right.

'What did you say, sweetie?'

I licked some icing off my finger, trying to appear nonchalant as my heart started beating that little bit faster.

'Mummy, I asked what kind of operation you had on your tummy? It was an operation, wasn't it?'

Taking her by the hand and leading her away from the melee to a quiet corner of the hallway, I crouched down so our eyes were level and held her gently by the shoulder with one hand, taking over twirling her blonde curls with the other.

'People have operations when they have something wrong with them and they have a surgery to get it fixed. The doctor does it to make people better and, yes, I had one on my tummy. Why do you want to know?'

I tried to keep my voice level. I'd dreaded these questions since Faith had been a baby in my arms. But I took a deep breath and tried to stay calm, reminding myself they might not be coming now.

'Why did you have an operation on your tummy, Mummy, what was wrong with it? Someone at school told me you had an operation for something but I can't remember what it's called.'

Her wide eyes stared so innocently at me as she tried to remember; looking into them, I fought to hold back the tears. This wasn't about me; it was about Faith. Faith was six years, five hours and thirty-seven minutes old and the question I'd hoped would wait until her teenage years had surfaced just after a room full of all her friends had sung her happy birthday.

'Shell, Faith, what are you doing? Everyone's in here…'

Hugh could see by my face and Faith's concentration that we were in the middle of something. Something big.

'We'll be in in a minute, Hugh, won't we, Faith? We're just having a quick chat about Mummy's operation on her tummy.'

Hugh took the cue and as I nodded to tell him I was handling it, he disappeared back round the corner. I took a deep breath, sat on the floor and pulled Faith onto my lap.

'Mummy has something in me that could make me sick, so I had an operation to make sure I won't get sick.'

'The one on your tummy?'

'Yes, Faith, the operation on my tummy was to make sure I won't get sick so we can have tonnes of birthday cakes and parties together every year…'

I could hear my voice catching, so took a deep breath and held her close.

'Mummy, will I get sick?'

Holding her head under my chin as silent tears streamed down my face, I didn't know what to say. I couldn't lie, but the truth was too enormous.

'We all might get sick, Faith; no one knows, but when you get older we can make sure you don't get sick either... Does that make sense?'

'Will I have to have an operation?'

'I don't know, sweetie, but if you do, I'll be with you every step of the way, is that OK?'

'OK, I love you, Mummy.'

And with that she climbed off my lap and ran back to her friends. Seconds later, as my tears kept falling, I could hear peals of her laughter echoing around the house. Hugh came looking for me a minute later. He sat down beside me on the floor as I explained tearfully the conversation Faith and I had just had.

'You've done it, Shell, that's the first conversation over with. You've explained BRCA in terms she understands and as she gets older we'll explain it in more detail.'

I opened my mouth to tell Hugh I felt awful, that it was all my fault, that I'd potentially ruined her life and that I'd never forgive myself, but something stopped me. Whether it was the fact it was Faith's birthday or the fact the house was filled with her friends, my friends, laughter and a tonne of love – whatever the reason, I stopped and nodded. Hugh was right.

There's so much about these circumstances I can't change but how Faith finds out and how she feels about it I can still fix. And while we won't know the outcome for at least another twelve years, until then I can fill her world with love and happiness.

Rising to my feet, squaring my shoulders and reaching for Hugh's hand, we both returned to the party. To love. To happiness and to the future.

THE END

Dealing with It: Finding What Works

Having battled with weight during my time in Liberty X and after training as a personal trainer in 2011, working out has been a lifeline for me for almost a decade. From receiving my BRCA results to living in menopause, working out, building up a sweat and aching afterwards has been a saviour for me.

I know it's not for everyone but trust me when I tell you, no one ever regrets a workout. And if you're reading this, thinking you hate exercise, you most likely haven't found the right kind yet, so don't give up. Whether that's a run in the park, a swim or some time in the gym, persevere and try different sports and classes until you find the one you like. I've always needed my gym time, but never more so than in menopause; it's literally become a tonic for me, and I wish the NHS could prescribe it for every single menopausal woman in the UK.

When you exercise, your body releases chemicals called endorphins. These endorphins interact with brain receptors, which trigger a feeling of happiness and contentedness in the brain, and never more so than in menopause do we need those happy hormones.

I try and stay emotionally strong as I experience menopause

but, even being a strong person, I'm totally weak at times – sometimes it's when I've ranted at the kids, other times it's when I've felt so low that I can't even get out of bed. Whatever the feeling, when menopause emotions get the better of me, the gym helps me by letting me forget. It's a distraction; whether I'm counting reps and sets or whether I'm so exhausted my mind is just filled with running one more mile, building up a sweat is a saviour to me.

When I get so low I feel like I can't breathe, like I'm drowning, or when the bleakness owns me, sweating it out helps. It takes my mind off it in that moment and the feel-good factor after a workout helps lift the darkness, even just a little. In those moments when I can't even tell myself that it'll pass, putting on my trainers and getting a sweat going makes all the difference. Don't get me wrong, it's not like I lace up my trainers happily every time – sometimes it's a real wrench to get out there and get going, but within a few minutes of getting my blood pumping, I'm always glad I've done it.

Without exercise, I don't know where I'd be. It's been my own kind of therapy, and women who stop me in the street have told me it's theirs too. Everyone has that different thing, that activity, person, place or time that they know can bring them round from the pit of despair and mine's the gym or the tarmac.

I know if I work out enough I'll look good and I know if I look good I'll feel good, but it's way more than that. I'm someone to everyone else – mum, wife, Michelle, sister, daughter – but in the gym the moment is just for me and I'm able to forget about everything. Everything I'm not, everything I can't do. Doing reps and sets, I don't think about work, the kids, the BRCA2 gene, the menopause. I think about pushing myself harder and faster. Nothing matters in the times I'm working out and that space I can create in my head every day is vital for me.

While the gym is definitely my safe haven and has saved me from myself constantly, it's also important to work out and exercise and stay healthy in menopause for physical as well as mental reasons. With a change in hormones in menopause, metabolism slows down; menopausal women don't need as many calories as pre-menopausal women but I don't know anyone – myself included – who's adjusted their diet to eat less in menopause, which is why working out is a must to help prevent the weight gain so many menopausal women fall prey to. Weight gain is included in plenty of symptom lists if you search for the menopause on the internet but it doesn't have to be.

If you're reading this and are one of millions of women across the UK who have gained weight since they went into menopause, the double whammy I'm about to deliver might not make you feel any better initially but bear with me… Losing weight in menopause takes longer than normal too. So not only are you more prone to weight gain, you'll also find it harder to lose.

Metabolic changes during this time make women's body's more sensitive to carbohydrate and sugars, which can mean you become more insulin-resistant. So if you've already got lots of carbs and sugars in your diet, you're unknowingly promoting fat storage, which is tough to shift.

Experts suggest women in menopause need around 200 calories a day less than women in their twenties. That's 1,400 calories a week to try and cut out from your diet. I know that, for me, that is a really unrealistic target, so my solution is to work out more instead.

Muscle mass also decreases when you're in menopause, resulting in a much lower resting metabolic rate than that of someone in their twenties or thirties. So working out helps not only to burn off the extra calories you might be consuming but no longer needing, but also to delay the inevitable muscle loss that comes with that stage in life.

Add in the fact that the majority of the UK population gets less active when they get older and you've got a recipe for menopausal weight gain which will be difficult to shift, potentially making you feel unhappy with your reflection and leaving you feeling down about everything.

Menopausal weight gain really is a vicious cycle which is another reason why exercise can become your 'go to' if you let it. Statistics show menopausal women are at a higher risk of heart disease and getting the heart pumping will reduce your risks – it won't only make you feel and look good, it'll keep your ticker healthy too.

While it'd be nice to think weight gain and metabolism are the only physical changes during menopause, there's also skin dryness, lack of sleep, night sweats, increased risk of osteoporosis… it's a long and delightful list of symptoms, and while the extent to which the symptoms affect anyone will vary from person to person, as a general rule of thumb, the best way of describing it is to say that everything – Every. Single. Thing. – is harder in menopause.

And while I know I'm a gym evangelist, getting out in the fresh air and raising your heart rate, even if it's just for a few minutes a day, will help counteract a lot of these symptoms. Not to mention the fact that time outdoors every day has been proven in numerous global studies to protect mental health.

If you're struggling to sleep, working out or doing some sport will mean you're physically exhausted and more likely to drop off. Weight-bearing exercises, walking, squats holding a couple of bags of sugar or press-ups will help bone density and keep bones strong, reducing the risk of developing osteoporosis. A US study of 60,000 post-menopausal women found a brisk walk four or more times per week lowered the risk of hip fractures when compared to a control group.

While I know it sounds like a sales pitch, there's nothing that won't be improved in menopause by starting to work out or finding a regular exercise you enjoy doing.

It might sound counterintuitive, but building up a sweat – however you choose to do it – will also help with the hot flushes that seem to be the hardest symptom to cope with, if the women who stop me in the street are anything to go by. Researchers at the Research Institute for Sport and Exercise Sciences at Liverpool John Moores University found women in menopause who undertook regular workouts for a period of four months reduced the frequency and intensity of their hot flushes. So if hot flushes are holding you back, start working out and you can reduce the severity of them, which might make them more manageable and easier to live with.

The average woman gains between 5lb and 7lb during menopause – I know I certainly gained around that and I have to work hard to keep it off – but whatever you choose to do and however you choose to exercise, your menopausal symptoms and your energy levels will all improve if you get the blood flowing a few times a week.

If you're already sporty, or if you walk the dog or run, then great, keep doing what you're doing and maybe increase the length of time or frequency of it, but if you're a novice or starting out with exercise, I've devised a menopause-friendly workout which can help you lose weight, get fit, reduce your risk of osteoporosis and improve the symptoms you're living with.

Take it easy to begin with and if you have any other medical conditions, please consult a doctor before you give this a go.

Menopause Workout

DAY 1:   CIRCUIT

Warm-up
3–5 minutes of jumping jacks or running on the spot

Main Phase
4–6 rounds (depending on fitness level) – 45 seconds for each exercise, 15 seconds' rest between each exercise

1–2 minutes' rest (depending on fitness level) between each round

1. Lunges
2. Press-ups (half or normal, depending on fitness level)
3. High knees
4. Plank (hold as long as you can, keep getting up within the 45 seconds)
5. Squats (or jumping squats, depending on fitness level)
6. Bicep curl (or shoulder press without weight while jogging on the spot)

Cool-down / Abs and Bums
5 minutes

1. Glute kickbacks
2. Crunches
3. Front leg raises

> Circuit training is about building strength and toning.
> Day 1 will help work towards reducing the risk of
> injury if, like me, you're prone to back pain or twists
> since entering menopause.

DAY 2: CARDIO

Warm-up
3–5 minutes of jumping jacks or running on the spot

Main Phase
Find a nearby hill.

1. Power-walk up for 60 seconds
2. Walk down
3. Run up it as fast as you can for 30 seconds
4. Walk down

Rest when needed and repeat as many times as you
can in 30 minutes.

Cool-down / Abs and Bums
5 minutes

1. Glute kickbacks
2. Crunches
3. Front leg raises

Cardio workouts reduce stress levels and increase bone density, which is vital in menopause, when osteoporosis is a risk. They also improve sleep patterns and quality of sleep, in addition to temporarily relieving anxiety, so whatever your symptoms, cardio can help.

DAY 3: CIRCUIT

Warm-up
3–5 minutes of jumping jacks or running on the spot

Main Phase
4–6 rounds (depending on fitness level) – 45 seconds for each exercise, 15 seconds' rest between each exercise

1–2 minutes' rest (depending on fitness level) between each round

1. Side lunges
2. Press-ups (half or normal, depending on fitness level)
3. Squats or kick-outs
4. Tricep dips
5. Jumping jacks
6. Squat and hold (20 seconds, rest for 5 seconds and back for another 20 seconds)

Cool-down / Abs and Bums
5–8 minutes

1. Outer thigh raises
2. Bicycle crunches
3. Plank (hold as long as you can, keep getting up within the 45 seconds)

DAY 4: CARDIO

Warm-up
3–5 minutes of jumping jacks or running on the spot

Main Phase
Find a street full of lamp posts.

1. Power-walk to the first one
2. Run as fast as you can to the next
3. Gentle walk to the next
4. Turn around and repeat

Rest when needed and repeat as many times as you can in 30 minutes.

Cool-down / Abs and Bums
5 minutes

1. Glute kickbacks
2. Crunches
3. Front leg raises

DAY 5: CIRCUIT

Warm-up
3–5 minutes of jumping jacks or running on the spot

Main Phase
4–6 rounds (depending on fitness level) – 45 seconds for each exercise, 15 seconds' rest between each exercise

1–2 minutes' rest (depending on fitness level) between each round

1. Jumping squats (or normal squats if a beginner)
2. Press-ups (half or normal, depending on fitness level)
3. Jump rope
4. Lunges
5. Shoulder press (if using no weight, jog on the spot while elevating arms)
6. Plank (hold as long as you can, keep getting up within the 45 seconds)

Cool-down / Abs and Bums
5-8 minutes

1. Outer thigh raises
2. Bicycle crunches
3. Plank (hold as long as you can, keep getting up within the 45 seconds)

DAY 6:   ACTIVE REST DAY

> Do something with the family, like:
>
> Gentle bike ride
> Go swimming
> Walk round the park and race each other at
> different points
> Long walk
> Game of tennis

DAY 7:   REST DAY

My Menopause Musings

While the benefits of working out in menopause are plentiful, if working out doesn't make you as happy as it makes me, find something that does, whether it's a hobby you used to have as a child, like art, or whether it's gardening or volunteering for a local charity.

In menopause, it's so easy to get lost and feel like you're drowning. Some days it's all I can do to get through unscathed and some days I don't think I can find the time for a workout, but setting aside some time every day just for you will do wonders for your emotional well-being during this time.

Whether it's reading a good book or calling a friend for a chat, as women we're not always best at prioritising our needs over those of our family or friends or employers, but relaxing and doing something you enjoy will protect your metal health as you try and navigate your way through menopause.

If you struggle to relax, there are plenty of mindfulness apps you can try for free. What's important is that you set aside some time daily where you are priority number one and nothing and no one else can interfere. It doesn't have to be long. Half an hour – twenty minutes, if that's all you can spare – will make a world of difference.

While my family is on this journey with me, I'm a better wife and mother on the days where I prioritise myself a little bit at the start or end of the day, so it's not just you who will benefit if you begin to take better care of yourself.

Eat Your Way to a Healthy Menopause

While I know working out has helped me cope with the emotional and physical fallout of being in menopause, my diet has always been important to me and never more so than at this time.

From wanting to come back from the hospital to start eating better, to making sure I eat with my husband round the table every night so we can keep a dialogue about everything going, food isn't just fuel for me, it's more than that. Eating right in menopause keeps my skin clear, my bones strong, my body nourished and my stomach full.

Hugh has always been into eating healthy and while I've admitted to bingeing sometimes and we always binge together on a Sunday, I work at my best and my body functions at its best when it's nourished with a healthy balance of home-made foods with plenty of nutrients, vitamins and minerals.

I'm not prescriptive about my diet, but over the years on this path I've learned which foods work for me and which ones don't. Eating right, eating clean and eating natural foods has always helped me combat my symptoms of the menopause, from a lack of energy to dry skin. Hugh and I are both personal trainers and while there's a nutrition section in the personal training course, we're both fans of clean, light, healthy meals, which don't leave us feeling lethargic and sleepy while we digest them.

Every menopause journey is different but mine is a time-poor one. I have the kids during the day with no childcare and I work a lot of evenings and weekends. I don't have the time to cook meals that take hours, so I try and shop for fresh ingredients and always in season – mostly because it makes them more wallet-friendly.

On an average week, my diet consists of things like vegetables and egg whites in an omelette for breakfast, asparagus if it's in season, as it's a natural diuretic and helps water leave the system. I have spinach on the side or in the omelette and then cheese. I've never been someone who sees fat as the enemy and I choose to get my fats from things like cheese rather than egg yolks.

I'll have a shake mid-morning with protein powder and coffee and I blend it up like an iced mocha. It fills a hole and the protein powder helps to repair and build muscles if I've had a particularly tough session at the gym.

Lunch is usually an oversized salad or vegetables or a ratatouille and then a protein bar in the afternoon.

For dinner, Hugh and I eat after the kids are in bed and we have something different every night. I'll make a healthy shepherd's pie – instead of potato, it'll be mashed up vegetables, and instead of beef mince, it'll be turkey mince.

Below is a typical week's food intake for me – it's menopause-friendly, with lots of ingredients which will help with symptoms from the inside out.

MONDAY

Breakfast

Smoked Salmon and Scrambled Eggs with Fruit on the Side

Serves 1

INGREDIENTS

> 1-calorie cooking spray
>
> 4 free-range egg whites
>
> 2 slices of rye bread
>
> 120g smoked salmon
>
> 2 lemon segments
>
> Freshly ground black pepper, to taste
>
> ½ grapefruit or 1 apple

METHOD

Scramble the egg whites in a pan using 1-calorie cooking spray, stirring gently until fluffy and cooked through.

Meanwhile, toast the rye bread.

Once the toast is ready, load it onto a plate and split the smoked salmon between the two slices. Squeeze lemon juice over the salmon.

Serve the scrambled eggs, either on top of the toast or on the side. Add a grind of black pepper over both the salmon and the eggs.

Follow your breakfast with ½ grapefruit or 1 small apple if you'd like, and a large glass of water.

Mid-morning Snack
Blueberry Smoothie

Serves 1

INGREDIENTS

1 cup frozen blueberries
100ml almond milk

METHOD

In a blender or using a stick blender, pulse and mix the frozen blueberries with the almond milk to the desired consistency.

I like mine completely smooth, but if you want some bites of blueberry in there just blend for a shorter time.

Strain into a glass and drink while ice cold.

Lunch
Prawn Cucumber Boats with Lentils

Serves 2

INGREDIENTS

1 cup red lentils
1 large, thick cucumber
4 cherry tomatoes
½ medium avocado
Squeeze of lime
Heinz Salad Cream 70% Less Fat
120–150g prawns, cooked and peeled
2 sweet red peppers, diced
¼ medium white onion, diced
Freshly ground black pepper, to taste

METHOD

Simmer the lentils in a pan of boiling water for 15 minutes or until cooked through. Make sure you use a big enough pan, as the lentils will double in size.

Cut the cucumber into two lengthways, and scoop out the seeds so your halves resemble little boats.

Halve the cherry tomatoes and put to one side.

Scoop out the avocado half and slice it, covering the slices with a squeeze of lime juice to stop them going brown.

In a bowl, add the salad cream together with the prawns, peppers and onion. Mix and season with pepper to taste.

Pack the cucumber boats with your prawn mixture and place slices of avocado on top.

Serve with the lentils and cherry tomatoes on the side and a big glass of water.

Mid-afternoon Snack
125–150g edamame / 1 × 40g bag of popcorn

Serves 1

Health food shops and most supermarkets serve nude popcorn, which has mild salt on it.

If you prefer edamame and can't buy it fresh from your local supermarket, it's available frozen from most supermarkets. Follow the pack instructions to cook it.

Dinner
Turkey Mince Shepherd's Pie with Vegetable Topping

Serves 2

INGREDIENTS

> 1-calorie cooking spray
> 300g lean turkey mince
> 1 large white onion, diced
> 4 cups frozen mixed veg
> 4 tsp low-salt gravy granules

METHOD

Preheat the oven at 200°C/400°F/Gas mark 6.

Boil the vegetables until cooked through, don't cook them al dente as you'll be using this for your topping. Drain them and put to one side.

Cook the mince and onion in a saucepan with 1-calorie spray until browning and thoroughly cooked through.

Make the gravy as per the pack instructions and add to the turkey and onion. Cook for another 10 minutes.

Place the turkey mince mix into a deep oven dish.

Mash the mixed vegetables with a potato masher – you won't get the same consistency as mash, but that's OK, you want some chunks in it.

Spread the layer of mashed vegetable over the turkey mixture and bake in the oven for around 15 to 20 minutes, or until the mashed vegetables start to brown at the edges.

This dish can be made ahead and frozen for ease, or you can have some the following day for lunch.

Serve with a large glass of water.

TUESDAY

Breakfast
Boiled Eggs and Toast with Grapefruit Side

Serves 1

INGREDIENTS

> 2 free-range eggs
> 2 slices of wholegrain or rye bread
> Low-sodium salt and freshly ground black pepper, to taste
> ½ grapefruit

METHOD

Boil the eggs in a pan of boiling water. Cook for 6 minutes for soft-boiled or 8 minutes for hard-boiled.

Toast the bread.

Serve the eggs in eggcups with a dash of salt and black pepper, to taste.

Follow the eggs with a ½ grapefruit, and a large glass of water.

Mid-morning Snack
Cottage Cheese and Apple

Serves 1

INGREDIENTS

> 150g low-fat cottage cheese
> 1 small apple

METHOD

Chop the apple into chunks – I prefer them diced quite small, whatever your preference.

Mix gently with cottage cheese.

Serve with a large glass of water.

Lunch
Chicken and Avocado Salad

Serves 1

INGREDIENTS

> 120–150g roast chicken breast, skin removed
> ½ medium avocado
> Squeeze of lime
> 1 little gem lettuce
> ¼ cup red or white onion, diced
> ½ cup sweetcorn
> ½ cup red pepper, diced
> 1 tbsp Heinz Salad Cream 70% Less Fat
> Freshly ground black pepper, plus extra to taste

METHOD

Tear up the chicken into long, chunky pieces and put into a large mixing bowl.

Slice the avocado or cut into chunks, squeeze over a bit of lime juice to stop it going brown and put it to one side.

Slice the lettuce into ribbons and add to the bowl of chicken.

Add the onion, sweetcorn and peppers to the bowl with the salad cream, and mix lightly. Add a few turns of the pepper mill.

Place the avocado on top and add more black pepper to taste. Serve with a large glass of water

Mid-afternoon Snack
100g of shop-bought jerky/biltong

Dinner
Stuffed, Baked Sweet Potato

Serves 1
For this recipe, you will need to choose some protein, which should already be cooked and finely chopped – you can use prawns, chicken, tuna in spring water, turkey, any kind of protein as long as it's lean.

INGREDIENTS

1 large sweet potato
120–150g of your chosen protein (see above)
½ cup no-added-sugar salsa
1 tsp pine nuts

Freshly ground black pepper

30g reduced-fat mozzarella, grated

METHOD

Bake the sweet potato in a preheated oven (200°C/400°F /Gas mark 6) for 35–40 minutes, until cooked. Leave the oven on, as you will be returning the potato to it shortly.

Mix your protein, salsa and pine nuts together, ensuring everything is mixed in with a few turns of the pepper mill.

Cut the baked sweet potato in half (take care, it will be hot from the oven!) and place the two portions so the inside of the potato is facing up on a baking tray.

Add the protein mix to the tops of the potato halves, packing on as much as you can before sprinkling the mozzarella over them.

Return to the oven and bake for a further 10–12 minutes until the mozzarella begins to brown.

WEDNESDAY

Breakfast
Turkey Rashers, Eggs and Grapefruit

Serves 1

INGREDIENTS

½ pack turkey rashers

1 free-range egg

1-calorie cooking spray

½ grapefruit

METHOD

Cook the turkey rashers under a hot grill for 3–4 minutes, turning every two minutes until thoroughly cooked.

Fry the egg in a frying pan using the cooking spray.

Serve the turkey and eggs with the grapefruit and a large glass of water.

Mid-morning Snack
Greek Yoghurt and Berries

Serves 1

INGREDIENTS

150g Total 0% Fat Greek Yoghurt
½ cup frozen berries of your choice

METHOD

Take the berries out of the freezer in the morning and allow them to sit until they reach room temperature.

Mix with the Greek yoghurt.

Serve with a large glass of water.

Lunch
Turkey Lettuce Wrap and Jersey Potatoes

Serves 1

INGREDIENTS

200g Jersey new potatoes
Pinch of low-sodium salt
1 beef tomato, diced

¼ cup red onion, diced
150g pre-cooked chicken or roast turkey breast,
sliced without the skin
¼ cup tinned kidney beans, drained
1 tsp lemon juice
1 tsp balsamic vinegar
freshly ground black pepper and low-sodium salt,
to taste
2 large lettuce leaves of your choice

METHOD

Cook the potatoes in a pan of lightly salted boiling water for 15 minutes or until tender.

Mix the tomato and onion together in a bowl.

Shred the roasted chicken or turkey into the tomato and onion mix, and add the kidney beans.

Dress the entire mixture including the potatoes with the lemon juice and balsamic vinegar, adding pepper and salt to taste.

Spoon the mixture gently into the middle of the lettuce leaves, and wrap the leaves over, burrito-style.

Serve with a large glass of water.

Mid-afternoon Snack
Blueberry, Cottage Cheese and Peanut Butter Smoothie

Serves 1

INGREDIENTS

> 1 cup cold water
> 1 cup ice
> ½ cup fresh or frozen blueberries
> ½ cup low-fat cottage cheese
> 1 tsp no-added-sugar peanut butter
> Sugar substitute such as stevia or agave, to taste

METHOD

Using a blender, Nutribullet or stick blender, blitz all the ingredients until frothy and blended, which should take around 30–40 seconds.

Serve immediately while still cold.

Dinner
Ham Pots and Sweet Potato Wedges

Serves 1

INGREDIENTS

> 1 large sweet potato
> Splash of olive oil
> Sprinkle of sea salt
> 1-calorie cooking spray
> 4 slices ham
> 2 free-range eggs
> ¼ cup low-fat Cheddar cheese, grated
> 1 cup mixed salad

METHOD

Preheat the oven at 200°C/400°F/Gas mark 6.

Cut the sweet potato into quarters lengthways, and then cut those lengths in half, so you end up with eight wedges.

Put the wedges on a baking tray, and splash with oil and sprinkle with salt. Bake for 35–40 minutes, turning regularly during the cooking process.

Take a Yorkshire pudding tray or muffin tin and spray with cooking spray. Place the sliced ham around on the bottom and around the sides of two of the pudding moulds, with a little overlap of slices.

Gently break an egg into each lined mould, being careful not to allow them to spill over the edges. If there's ham left overlapping the edges of the mould, gently fold it back on top of the egg, taking care not to break the yolk.

Lightly sprinkle over the grated cheese.

Reduce the oven temperature to 190°C/375°F/Gas mark 5 and bake for 15–18 minutes.

Remove the ham pots from the oven and leave to cool for 3–4 minutes, while you plate up your salad and add the wedges to it.

Gently run a knife around the edge of the ham, ensuring it's loose, and spoon your ham pots onto your mixed salad.

Serve with a large glass of water.

THURSDAY

Breakfast
Vegetable and Fruit Smoothie

Serves 1

INGREDIENTS

> 1 cup frozen berries of your choice
> ½ cup raw spinach
> 100g Total 0% Fat Greek Yoghurt
> ½ cup no-added-sugar almond milk or skimmed
> cow's milk
> 2 heaped tsp Options hot chocolate – flavour of
> your choice
> Sugar substitute such as stevia or Splenda, to taste
> 1 cup ice

METHOD

Using a blender, Nutribullet or stick blender, blitz all the ingredients until frothy and blended, which should take around 30–40 seconds.

Serve immediately while still cold.

Mid-morning Snack
Small banana, dipped into 1 tsp no-added-sugar peanut butter

Lunch
Tuna and Bean Fishcake

Serves 1

INGREDIENTS

       1 can tuna in spring water

       ¼ cup red or white onion, diced

       ¼ cup tinned chopped tomatoes

       ¼ cup tinned kidney beans, drained

       1 free-range egg

       1 tsp malt vinegar

       Freshly ground pepper and low-sodium salt, to taste

       4 stalks tender stem or purple sprouting broccoli

METHOD

Preheat the oven at 180°C/350°F/Gas mark 4.

Combine the tuna, onion and tomatoes in a mixing bowl.

Gently mash the kidney beans with the back of a fork.

Whisk the egg in a separate bowl and add in the kidney beans, then stir the egg and beans into the tuna mixture.

Season with vinegar, salt and pepper, and combine the mix until the ingredients resemble a chunky paste – it'll be quite a wet consistency.

With clean, wet hands, gently shape the mixture into two fishcakes.

Bake in the oven for 20–25 minutes, gently turning them halfway through, until they are crispy on the outside.

Steam the tender stem or purple sprouting broccoli in a few tablespoons of water until cooked but still al dente.

Serve the fishcakes with the broccoli and a large glass of water.

Mid-afternoon Snack
2 boiled eggs

Dinner
Lean Steak and Courgette Chips

Serves 1

INGREDIENTS

2 courgettes – opt for the skinniest courgettes you can find, as the chips work better with more skin and less flesh
1-calorie cooking spray
120–150g lean steak
¼ cup Parmesan, finely grated

METHOD

Preheat the oven at 200°C/400°F/Gas mark 6.

Cut the courgettes into fine batons, so they're French fry width and size. Spray them with the cooking spray.

Sprinkle the Parmesan onto the base of a shallow dish, then roll the courgette batons gently in the cheese, ensuring they're coated and covered on all edges and sides.

Bake in the oven for 15–20 minutes, turning occasionally, until they start to brown and crisp up.

Meanwhile, fry the steak to your preference using the cooking spray and leave to rest until the courgette fries are cooked.

Serve with a large glass of water.

FRIDAY

Breakfast
Salmon Hash

Serves 1

INGREDIENTS

100g salmon, cooked and flaked or tinned in spring water

2 free-range egg whites

½ cup raw spinach

1 cup mushrooms, diced

4 cherry tomatoes, diced

Freshly ground pepper and low-sodium salt, to taste

Fresh parsley, to taste

1-calorie cooking spray

1 tsp lemon juice

METHOD

Combine all the ingredients except for the lemon juice in a large bowl, seasoning to taste.

Spray a frying pan with the cooking spray, and scramble the mixture over a medium heat for 5 minutes until cooked.

Season with a couple of extra turns of the pepper mill and add the lemon juice.

Serve with a large glass of water.

The salmon hash can also be placed in an ovenproof dish, lightly greased with cooking spray, and baked for a further 10 minutes, for a crispier texture, if desired.

Mid-morning Snack
1 apple and 1 orange

Lunch
Turkey and Avocado Roll-ups with Lentils

Serves 1

INGREDIENTS

> 1 pack turkey rashers
> 1-calorie cooking spray
> ½ medium avocado
> A couple of squeezes of lemon
> Cocktail sticks
> ½ cup red lentils
> Pinch of low-sodium salt
> ½ bag rocket leaves
> Freshly ground black pepper

METHOD

Fry the turkey rashers in the cooking spray until cooked but still pliable – keeping a lid on the pan during the frying process will retain moisture. Remove from the heat and place on a plate.

Cut the avocado into slices, then lay a slice on each rasher. Add a squeeze of lemon juice over the avocado slices for flavour and to stop them browning.

Starting at one end of the rasher, roll up the avocado inside the rasher and secure with a cocktail stick so it doesn't unravel.

Boil the lentils in lightly salted water for 15 minutes, but be sure to use a big enough pan, as they'll double in size.

Serve the turkey and avocado roll-ups on top of the lentils. Dress the rocket with another squeeze of lemon juice and the black pepper, to taste, and serve on the side.

Serve with a large glass of water.

Mid-afternoon Snack
Handful of non-roasted, non-flavoured almonds and cashews – 15–20 nuts is about the right portion size

Dinner
Red Pepper Quiche

Serves 1

INGREDIENTS

> 1 red pepper
> 4 free-range egg whites
> 1 whole free-range egg
> 3 cloves garlic, finely chopped
> ¼ cup low-fat Cheddar, grated
> ¼ cup spring onions, chopped
> Freshly ground black pepper and low-sodium salt
> ½ cup broccoli
> ½ cup asparagus

METHOD

Preheat the oven at 200°C/400°F/Gas mark 6.

Cut the pepper in half across the middle, rather than lengthways. Scoop out all the seeds. Cut off the stalk from the top and place both halves on a baking tray on baking parchment, cut side up.

Mix together thoroughly the egg whites, whole egg, garlic, half the cheese and the spring onions. Season with salt and pepper.

Spoon the mixture into the red pepper cups and sprinkle the remaining cheese on top of the 'quiches'.

Bake for 15–20 minutes.

While the quiches are in the oven (about 10 minutes into baking), steam the broccoli and asparagus until cooked but still firm to the touch.

Do the 'wobble test' on the quiche after the first 15 minutes; if there is no wobble when you gently prod the peppers, the egg is thoroughly cooked.

Serve the quiches with the steamed vegetables and a large glass of water.

SATURDAY

Breakfast
Banana Nut Crunch Greek Yoghurt

Serves 1

INGREDIENTS

> 1 cup Total 0% Fat Greek Yoghurt
> 1 tbsp no-added-sugar crunchy peanut or almond butter
> ½ medium banana

METHOD

Without mixing it in completely, swirl the nut butter through the Greek yoghurt to create a rippled effect.

Slice the banana and lay it on top of the yoghurt.

Serve with a large glass of water.

Mid-morning Snack

Protein bar – make sure it contains less than 3g of sugar and fewer than 200 calories

Lunch

Protein Skewers and Sweet Potato

Serves 1

INGREDIENTS

1 medium sweet potato

120–150g of boneless, skinless chicken or lean beef or white fish

1 slice pineapple

1 red pepper

½ red onion

Bamboo skewers

1-calorie cooking spray

½ tsp ground ginger

¼ tsp chilli powder (optional)

Pinch of low-sodium salt

½ bag rocket leaves

METHOD

Preheat the oven at 180°C/350°F/Gas mark 4.

Bake the whole sweet potato in the pre-heated oven for 35–40 minutes or until cooked through.

Meanwhile, cut the meat or fish, pineapple, pepper and onion into thumb-size chunks or cubes, making sure they're all roughly the same size, so they'll all cook at the same time.

Slide the protein, pineapple, pepper and onion onto the skewers, alternating them, so you have the same amount of everything on a skewer.

Spray the skewers evenly with the cooking spray.

Mix together the ground ginger and chilli, if using, with a pinch of salt. Dust over the skewers, ensuring even coverage.

Place the skewers on a baking tray and bake in the oven (still set to 180°C/350°F/Gas mark 4) for 15 minutes, or until golden brown and cooked. Once you start to smell the ginger and chilli they're not far from being finished.

Serve the potato and skewers with half a bag of rocket and a large glass of water.

Mid-afternoon Snack
4–5 celery sticks dipped into 1 tsp no-added-sugar peanut or almond butter

Dinner
Turkey and Courgette Spaghetti

Serves 1

INGREDIENTS

      120–150g turkey mince

      1-calorie cooking spray

      ½ cup white onion, diced

      1 cup tinned tomatoes, no added sugar

      1 tsp tomato puree

      300g courgettes, grated into spaghetti-like strips (if you have a spiraliser, use that; if not, use a coarse grater or slice as thinly as possible)

      2 cloves garlic, finely chopped

      1 tsp herbs of your choice – rosemary, mixed herbs and oregano work well

      Pinch of low-sodium salt

      ¼ cup Parmesan cheese, finely grated

METHOD

Cook the mince in a saucepan with the cooking spray. When almost cooked but not yet browned, add in the onion, tomatoes and puree, stir and simmer for around 4 minutes.

Spray a separate pan with cooking spray, and sauté the courgette spaghetti with the garlic, herbs and salt until the spaghetti is slightly wilted – this should take 3–5 minutes.

Place the courgette spaghetti onto a plate, spoon the mince on top and sprinkle with Parmesan.

Serve with a large glass of water.

SUNDAY

Breakfast
Greek Yoghurt Bowl

Serves 1

INGREDIENTS

> 170g Total 0% Fat Greek Yoghurt
> 1 apple, diced
> 4 walnuts, chopped
> 1 tsp honey or sugar-free jam

METHOD

Lightly combine the yoghurt, apple and walnuts.

Warm the honey or jam in a microwave for 10 seconds, then drizzle over the yoghurt mixture.

Serve with a large glass of water.

Mid-morning Snack
Protein Shake with Banana

Serves 1

INGREDIENTS

> 1 scoop of protein powder – the powders come in tonnes of flavours, from cinnamon and chocolate to fruits, so pick whichever flavour you prefer
> 1 medium banana
> 50ml cold water
> 1 handful of ice
> 100ml unsweetened almond milk or skimmed cow's milk

METHOD

Using a blender, Nutribullet or stick blender, blitz all the ingredients until frothy and blended, which should take around 30–40 seconds.

Lunch
Omelette with Avocado

Serves 2

INGREDIENTS

1-calorie cooking spray
¼ cup mushrooms, diced
½ red onion, diced
1 tsp smoked paprika
1 cup spinach, washed
4 free-range egg whites
1 whole free-range egg
½ medium avocado
1 tsp lime juice
½ bag mixed salad

METHOD

Spray a frying pan with cooking spray and place over a medium heat. Gently fry the mushrooms and onions with the smoked paprika for a couple of minutes, before adding the spinach and allowing to soften.

Whisk the egg whites and whole eggs together until light and fluffy, then add to the mushroom and spinach mixture in the frying pan. Swirl so the mixture coats the bottom of the pan.

Gently fork in the edge of the egg mixture, swirling again as you go so the runny parts of the egg mixture continues to coat the bottom of the pan.

When there's no more runny egg to swirl, using a fish slice or large spatula, flip one half of the omelette onto the other half, so it looks like a half moon in the pan.

Place a lid on top and cook for a further 2–3 minutes.

Slice the avocado and sprinkle with the lime juice to stop it going brown.

Place the omelette on top of the mixed salad, with the avocado on the side.

Serve with a large glass of water.

Mid-afternoon Snack
Protein bar – make sure it contains less than 3g of sugar and fewer than 200 calories

Dinner
Chicken Bake

Serves 2

INGREDIENTS

     1-calorie cooking spray
     300g chicken or white fish, skinless and boneless, diced into cubes
     1 cup coconut milk or skimmed cow's milk
     ½ tsp cumin
     1 clove of garlic, crushed

1 tbsp curry powder (optional)

1 white onion, diced

1½ red peppers, diced

2 cups broccoli, stems removed and cut into florets

1 cup low-fat mozzarella

Freshly ground black pepper, to taste

½ bag mixed green salad

METHOD

Preheat the oven at 200°C/400°F/Gas mark 6.

Spray an ovenproof frying pan with a little cooking spray and place over a medium heat.

Add the chicken or fish to the pan. As it starts to cook, add the milk, cumin, garlic and curry powder (if using).

Add the onion and pepper to the protein and continue to simmer.

Add the broccoli to the pan, then transfer it to the oven straight away and bake for 10 minutes.

Combine the grated mozzarella with the black pepper. Remove the pan from the oven, sprinkle the seasoned cheese over the top, then return to the oven and bake for a further 5–8 minutes, or until the top is melted and browned.

Serve with the mixed green salad and a large glass of water.

This dish can be refrigerated and eaten the next day, or frozen.

My Menopause Musings

There are plenty of foods that are menopause-friendly; some contain nutrients that have been proven to combat menopause symptoms, or some have naturally occurring oestrogen in them, which can help improve balance in the body.

Include any of the following twenty-three foods in your shopping basket and your menopausal body will be thanking you. Whether you eat them on their own or whether you start including them in recipes or changing up your regular meals with some new ingredients, they've all been scientifically proven to benefit you at this time in your life.

If some of them are foods you haven't tried before, give them a go. You'll be surprised at what your menopausal palate will enjoy.

If you've got any allergies or are on any other special diet, though, make sure you check with a health professional first.

VEGETABLE CARBOHYDRATES

While not all carbohydrates are created equal, there's a big advantage for the perimenopausal or menopausal woman to include carbohydrates in her diet. Hormone changes during menopause directly affect brain chemistry, specifically serotonin, which has been linked to dips in mood; when serotonin levels are low, we're also more likely to crave sugary things, whether that's chocolate or wine. But before you reach for something your waistline and your brain chemistry will regret in the long term, think about carbs instead. Including a little carbohydrate in every meal could be all it takes for your body to raise its levels of serotonin and get you feeling more upbeat. Carbohydrates aren't only found in white bread and crisps, though; lentils, sweet potato, peas, corn, squash and beetroot are all high in carbohydrates and packed with plenty of other beneficial nutrients too. Next time you feel like you need a sugary boost, try some popcorn instead, and you'll soon see the difference.

NON-DAIRY CALCIUM

It won't come as a shock that weakening bone density and osteoporosis are big risks once you reach menopause, whatever age that is. While we should all be consuming plenty of calcium our entire lives, studies have found one out of every two menopausal women eat or drink less than the recommended daily amount of 500–1000mg calcium that is needed to reduce the risk of osteoporosis and slow the inevitable bone density issues which come with menopause. But increasing calcium intake doesn't have to mean increasing how much milk or cheese you consume – dark, leafy greens are an amazing source of calcium, not to mention fish such as sardines and salmon, and seeds such as sesame and chia.

VITAMIN D

While vitamin D is vital for general bone health, it's also needed to help the body absorb calcium. Low levels of vitamin D in menopausal women can lead to fatigue. While sunshine is one of the best forms of vitamin D, menopausal women often tend to be more concerned with ageing and skin protection, so your SPF could be reducing the amount of vitamin D you're absorbing from the sunshine. The good news is that there are plenty of dietary ways to get more of it into your system.

Oily fish such as fresh tuna and sardines are great sources of vitamin D, as are eggs and mushrooms. If those vitamin-D rich foods aren't to your liking, there are menopausal supplements available that mostly contain vitamin D – just make sure you speak to your health professional before starting any new course of supplements, especially if you have a pre-existing health condition.

WHOLE GRAINS

Women not yet in menopause have a lower risk of getting heart disease than the rest of the UK population but unfortunately once menopause sets in, that risk increases and continues to climb as we age. While research is ongoing, it's believed that there's a link between reduced oestrogen in the body and increased risk of heart disease. There's also evidence to suggest that cholesterol levels and blood pressure increase in menopause, both of which can directly impact heart health. While exercising will definitely help reduce the risk of heart disease, there are dietary changes which can also help. Fruits, vegetables, whole grains, legumes and unsalted nuts can all help keep your heart healthy in menopause. Keep your diet rich in fibre and you'll be helping protect your most vital organ.

WATER

Vaginal dryness and dry skin are common in menopause, and while there are hormonal reasons for both of them, keeping your entire system as hydrated as possible will go some way to reducing these symptoms. Make sure you drink at least eight large glasses of water a day; if you're struggling to get them down, infuse your water with some fruit and herbs – lemon and ginger is lovely, as is cucumber, strawberry and mint. If you're drinking your eight glasses a day and feel like you're constantly on your way to the toilet, eat water-rich foods like cucumber and watermelon or add herbal teas and broths into your diet to up your water intake.

B VITAMINS AND PROTEIN

B vitamins are often referred to as the 'stress' vitamins, and a quick look at any menopausal supplement will show you they're included in practically every single one. Symptoms of vitamin B deficiency include tension, irritability, anxiety, poor concentration and lack of energy, all of which can be symptoms during menopause too. While there are lots of different types of B vitamins, all with different functions, some vitamin B-rich foods include peas, eggs, whole grains, rice, fish, tomatoes and broccoli. I'm a big fan of protein, and protein combined with vitamin B will help stabilise blood sugar levels too, which can help alleviate energy dips and mood swings. Protein energy bars often have B vitamins in them, but check the label before you buy.

FLAX SEEDS

Flax seeds (or linseeds) are packed with fibre, which has heart-protecting benefits, as well as lignans, an antioxidant which has been found to reduce symptoms of menopause. Lignans are oestrogen-like compounds, which can help balance hormone levels. A teaspoon ground into soaked oats or eaten as a snack once or twice a week could go some way to helping manage your symptoms of menopause, as well as providing valuable heart protection properties.

ALMONDS

Almonds are packed with tonnes of nutritional benefits; if you don't like the nuts themselves, there's also almond milk, which can be used in place of dairy milk. They're a great source of fat and a few every other day could help reduce the dry skin that so often comes with menopause. Almonds also contain heart-protecting magnesium, vitamin E and riboflavin. If you're opting for almond milk, though, make sure you seek out the unsweetened option.

EGGS

I'm a big fan of eggs and eat them every other day, although I reduce my consumption of the yolks by using egg whites more often than whole eggs. Eggs are packed with iron, which is great news, as studies have found lots of women in menopause can be iron-deficient without realising it. Eggs have vitamins D and B too, which help with energy levels and make sure bones stay strong, both vital for women in menopause. While I know free-range eggs are more expensive, go for the best-quality eggs you can afford, to pack an extra nutritional punch.

SOY

Soy contains plant oestrogens, so including it in your diet can help several symptoms of menopause. The largest study of its kind found two servings of 54mg daily reduced the frequency of hot flushes by just over 20 per cent and the severity of hot flushes by around 26 per cent. I include soy in my diet, but in its natural form, edamame, rather than in processed forms.

BRAIN FOODS

Blueberries have long been linked to a multitude of health benefits, from protecting brain function to reducing vision problems in older people, but a recent study from the US has found they could also protect against heart disease by lowering blood pressure, which can increase in menopausal women. Menopausal women in the US with high blood pressure were split into two groups, with half of them given a cup of blueberries every day for eight weeks and the other half given a placebo. At the end of the trial, blood pressure had decreased in all the women who consumed the blueberries. I include these delicious berries in my breakfasts, frozen and blitzed up in smoothies, and generally as a snack.

FIBRE, WATER AND PROTEIN

As I've already mentioned, weight gain is inevitable for lots of women in menopause, but the healthy trinity of fibre, water and protein can help you fill up quicker and stay full for longer through fewer calories. I'm a big fan of broccoli, which is packed with fibre and is an excellent addition to protein shakes and smoothies. I always make sure I have lean protein with my meals and plenty of water during the day. Some foods that contain all three include black beans, kidney beans and lentils. High-protein porridge will also give you a shot of all three and keep you full up.

FRUIT

While fruit is packed with nutrients, it's also pretty high in sugar, which won't help you lose any weight gained in menopause, despite how nutritious it is. There are low-sugar fruits though; I have a lot of grapefruit in my diet, and I also use avocado in lots of my meals – although it is used in savoury recipes, it is actually a fruit, one that is low in sugar and high in really good fats. Cranberries and raspberries are also low in sugar, and the latter is packed with fibre too. I avoid fruit juices, as they have a high sugar content and all the beneficial fibre of the fruit is lost when the fruit pulp is taken out. It's easy to add some low-sugar fruit into your breakfast or lunchtime and your waistline will thank you for it in the long run.

VEGETABLES

As my need for calories has decreased in menopause, I've been packing my mealtimes with vegetables for years now. Choosing the right ones can mean you meet your entire vitamin and nutrient needs while staying very healthy and avoiding too many calories. Broccoli, peas – whatever's seasonal is usually what ends up in my shopping basket. I always make sure I have plenty of frozen veg in the freezer to cook with too, whether it's for an omelette or a turkey shepherd's pie topping. There's not much you can't use vegetables in.

OMEGA 3 FOODS

Foods rich in omega 3, such as oily fish like salmon and mackerel, reduce the risk of high cholesterol, which is common after menopause. There's also evidence that including them in a balanced and healthy diet, along with regular exercise, could reduce the risk of heart disease, another condition linked to menopause. Omega 3 is also available in supplement form along with fish oil, but speak to your GP or health professional before you start taking any supplements, especially if you have a pre-existing condition.

PROTEIN-BOUND IODINE

It sounds like something you'd find in a laboratory, but protein-bound iodine can be found in cod, tinned tuna, cranberries and green beans. It's been found to help hormone production, which can be in free fall in menopause, and also helps general organ function and health.

IRON-RICH FOODS

During menopause, women are at an increased risk of anaemia, which means there are low levels of iron in the blood. Symptoms can be the same as menopause – lack of energy, insomnia, headaches – so it's important to include plenty of iron-rich foods in your diet. Red meat, such as steak, is a great source of iron, and eggs and leafy, green vegetables like kale, spinach and chard can help too. If you suspect you have anaemia in menopause, make an appointment with your GP or health professional, who'll be able to check your iron levels.

SWEET POTATO

Sweet potato is one of the highest sources of plant-based oestrogens. Like its flax seed cousin, it's packed with lignans and is a complex carbohydrate, which means it can boost energy levels. For some women, sweet potato can lessen the effect of reduced oestrogen in the body and combat tiredness, insomnia and dry skin.

BROCCOLI

I probably eat more broccoli than I do any other vegetable. In addition to the fact it's delicious, it's also incredibly versatile and I use it in everything from breakfasts to dinners. It's packed with calcium, which helps build strong bones, and contains phenolic compounds, which have been found in large-scale studies in the US to reduce the risk of heart disease and type two diabetes.

LEGUMES

Magnesium levels tend to decrease during menopause, resulting in lack of energy, headaches and poor sleep patterns. You can get magnesium into your diet through eating beans and lentils, which are also packed with heart-protecting fibre. I love kidney beans, and use them mashed in fishcakes and in wraps too.

RAW CARROTS

These orange sticks of goodness have long been heralded for their health benefits – they're packed with vitamins and minerals, including lutein, a carotenoid compound that can help improve dry skin and keep your heart healthy. They're also brimming with vitamins A and C, both of which have been found to deplete during menopause

FIGS

While they're not cheap even when in season, fresh figs (forget the dried ones) help lower blood pressure. It's worth remembering, however, that they're very high in sugar, so maybe limit yourself to a quarter of a cup a week.

GLUTEN-FREE GRAINS

While they're no doubt towards the top of the 'trendy' food lists, grains like brown rice, buckwheat, quinoa and millet are high in fibre and packed with protein and vitamins. There's evidence to suggest they can help with menopause symptoms but, regardless of that, they will help you feel fuller for longer, which could potentially reduce the risk of weight gain during menopause.

Thanks

While I've been fortunate enough not to endure any hot flushes so far, they're one of the most common menopausal symptoms, which is why I decided to use it as a title for this book. Are they in my future? Most likely, and they seem to be one of the more debilitating symptoms and are the hardest to live with. My mum still suffers from hot flushes and has to carry a fan with her everywhere. We've had to leave places before when she's been so hot, which has been embarrassing for her. Besides, without using the M word itself, if you say the words to anyone, they'll instantly know you're talking about menopause.

However this book ended up in your hands, I want to say thank you. Whether you've read it for you, or to learn more about something someone you love is going through, I'm grateful for the opportunity I've been given to share my story.

It's been six years I wouldn't ever want to repeat – my husband and children haven't made it out unscathed and it's changed us all irreversibly, but we're stronger for it. We appreciate more because of it and we're tighter thanks to it.

There's so much that needs to change in the menopause landscape in terms of understanding, and I hope by some small token I've been able to make a difference to the way it's talked about, thought about and spoken about.

I've spent years ashamed of my genetics. Those feelings of not being good enough or of being a failure because of my DNA are still with me and most likely will stay for a very long time. I'm trying to reframe my thoughts to feel differently, but it's not easy. Hugh reminds me all the time that none of this is my fault, but my body had the faulty gene and because of that I had to have the surgeries I've had. It's my body's fault I'm in menopause and so everything that goes along with that is my fault.

While Hugh would disagree with me, he'd agree whole-heartedly about the fact that my menopause has changed all our worlds. I don't know what the future holds for me – I know the symptoms I've spoken about are still there and I don't know if they'll ever go. I also don't know whether I've got different symptoms ahead of me.

I wouldn't be who I am without the unswerving and unending support my husband, Hugh, has given me every day since we got married. I wouldn't have learned so much about myself as a person and my capacity for love without my two incredible, funny, feisty, brave children, Faith and AJ. When you are old enough to read this and understand what mummy has written, I want you to know that, without your love and the strength you give me without even knowing it every single day, I may not have been able to carry on. I did this for you, for your dad, for us. And 'us' is all that matters to me. All three of you are my world. There is not one person I know better than you, Hugh, in every single way. You are everything!

I wouldn't have the moral compass I have if it wasn't for my mum and dad, who raised me right and encouraged me to set the bar high and never stop trying to reach it. You both, and David, have been the best family I could wish for. I do love you all, even if life has paved a different path where we are no longer all together, in my early memories we are – and they were happy. Special shout to my mummy, my friend my equal. Thank you for making me the person I am today I'm here because of you! And I love you (and angel) very much. Without my surgeon, Mr Sheridan, my journey would have been harder and his honesty – while occasionally upsetting me – has been something I've valued at every single turn.

I can't thank every single friend in my life, I've been blessed with so many beautiful souls and special people who have been there for me along the way. But may I thank especially my second family, Vivianna, (and Liz, of course) Troy, and mummy Silvana and Tony, David and Briony and my princess Aurora. Your continued love and support makes you my family.

And my actual second family, the Hanley's. You welcomed this crazy Geordie girl with open arms into your lives ten years ago. And you let me steal your Hughie away. You know how much I adore him, and adore you all for letting me have him!

My girls Rochelle and Victoria, without your help with Faith, AJ and my ever-hectic life and schedule … it would probably unravel at the seams! I really do look up to you both (even though I'm older) you are (not in this order) my eating, drinking, waking, gossiping, laughing workout bunnies! Love you both very much. Of course, Ben too! You and Hugh are the good ones. Me and Rochelle are very lucky women!

To new friends like all the Beeches Mums and my ladies Alex and Hayley, who have suffered more than their fair share of family tragedy and have both lit up my world and made me see it from angles I never knew existed. To old friends, Michelle, my longest-suffering friend lol. Even though we have not been as close through the last six years, the times we've had together are some of my fondest and happiest memories … love you babe and I'm always here for you, even 300 miles away.

Claire and Jimmy, your friendship to us both – especially in Vegas – has been much appreciated and we wish we could see more of you all.

Inanch and Penny, two of the most fearless, strong, generous women I know, with the most beautiful souls inside and out. And without whom I'd probably look like crap!

The Morocco girls, aka 'panto babes', we've shared so much over a short period of time – from a mountain in Morocco to a gossip over champagne – thank you for always being shoulders to cry on – literally!

Kirsty and your beautiful (crazy) wonderful family of children, dogs, pigs and ducks, lol for welcoming us into your lives over the last year. Again, not unaccustomed to life's challenges, but one of the strongest women I know.

How can I not mention my Liberty X peeps! Kelli, Jessica, Kevin and Tony. While we may not have been together much during the times I've written about in this book, you have all played a part in the times in my life that made me the woman I am today. You all know me well, and know how much I love life and live life to the full … and I have never had so much life and fun than I did with you guys. If I could do Liberty X all over again, I would. I miss all being together.

May I also take this time to thank the person who made this book actually happen … my wonderful manager, Ali, you have been more than a manager to me. You are one of my best friends. Hugh and the kids love you … and you are so much fun! I've had the best times with you and I'm sure many more to come! But under all the fun, you are my voice of reason and you keep me in line … much to Hugh's pleasure lol. Without you I'd still be dreaming of writing this book! Look at us, published book, babe! Cheers!

Clare – what can I say but thank you for being on this journey with me. It's been a rollercoaster at times but you have been amazing to work with, the late night WhatAapps, Facetimes and working around the kids' school times and holidays! Oh, the glamour and the reality. You helped me gather my thoughts and put this crazy journey into words.

Jo – thank you for your wisdom, calm and kind words and unfailing support – we did it!

Louise and all at Michael O'Mara Books – thank you for believing in me and letting me tell my story. Though difficult at times it's been an important step in my life. You made it all happen and I couldn't be prouder.

With the past behind me, the future in front of me and these pages almost finished, I've made some promises to myself too.

I've promised to be more open. I know some of the issues I've dealt with in the last few years might have had a lesser effect or might not have been so huge if I'd opened up and been honest about them, rather than trying to figure them out on my own.

I've promised to keep trying to change. All any of us can do is evolve if we want to keep moving forward and every behaviour I exhibit, every cross word, every confidence knock, I'll keep trying to learn from them to become a better person.

I've promised to be kinder to myself too. A lot of my behaviours have had hugely self-destructive elements to them. I've promised to try to start believing I am good enough, that I do deserve what I have and that I am worth something.

I've promised to be thankful. I mess up, I get things wrong and I'm not perfect, but I'm here. I wake up every morning and I'm cancer-free.

I'm Michelle Heaton and this has been my journey.

In loving memory of the beautiful Christina Earl,
taken from us far too soon.

You were a ray of sunshine on the darkest of days –
thank you for helping me make this book possible.

Index

(the initials MH refer to Michelle Heaton)